Noha Swilam

**Chemistry and Biology of Phenolics Isolated from Myricaria Germanica**

Noha Swilam

# Chemistry and Biology of Phenolics Isolated from Myricaria Germanica

Südwestdeutscher Verlag für Hochschulschriften

**Impressum / Imprint**

Bibliografische Information der Deutschen Nationalbibliothek: Die Deutsche Nationalbibliothek verzeichnet diese Publikation in der Deutschen Nationalbibliografie; detaillierte bibliografische Daten sind im Internet über http://dnb.d-nb.de abrufbar.

Alle in diesem Buch genannten Marken und Produktnamen unterliegen warenzeichen-, marken- oder patentrechtlichem Schutz bzw. sind Warenzeichen oder eingetragene Warenzeichen der jeweiligen Inhaber. Die Wiedergabe von Marken, Produktnamen, Gebrauchsnamen, Handelsnamen, Warenbezeichnungen u.s.w. in diesem Werk berechtigt auch ohne besondere Kennzeichnung nicht zu der Annahme, dass solche Namen im Sinne der Warenzeichen- und Markenschutzgesetzgebung als frei zu betrachten wären und daher von jedermann benutzt werden dürften.

Bibliographic information published by the Deutsche Nationalbibliothek: The Deutsche Nationalbibliothek lists this publication in the Deutsche Nationalbibliografie; detailed bibliographic data are available in the Internet at http://dnb.d-nb.de.
Any brand names and product names mentioned in this book are subject to trademark, brand or patent protection and are trademarks or registered trademarks of their respective holders. The use of brand names, product names, common names, trade names, product descriptions etc. even without a particular marking in this work is in no way to be construed to mean that such names may be regarded as unrestricted in respect of trademark and brand protection legislation and could thus be used by anyone.

Coverbild / Cover image: www.ingimage.com

Verlag / Publisher:
Südwestdeutscher Verlag für Hochschulschriften
ist ein Imprint der / is a trademark of
OmniScriptum GmbH & Co. KG
Heinrich-Böcking-Str. 6-8, 66121 Saarbrücken, Deutschland / Germany
Email: info@svh-verlag.de

Herstellung: siehe letzte Seite /
Printed at: see last page
**ISBN: 978-3-8381-3968-5**

Zugl. / Approved by: Greifswald, PH, Diss, 2014

Copyright © 2014 OmniScriptum GmbH & Co. KG
Alle Rechte vorbehalten. / All rights reserved. Saarbrücken 2014

**CONTENTS**

| | |
|---|---|
| LIST OF TABLES | VII |
| LIST OF FIGURES | VIII |
| LIST OF ABBREVIATION | XI |
| | Page |

| | | |
|---|---|---|
| 1 | INTRODUCTION ................................................................... | 1 |
| 2 | REVIEW OF LITERATURE ................................................. | 7 |
| | **2.1. BOTANY** ............................................................................ | 7 |
| | 2.1.1. Botanical description of the family Tamaricaceae............... | 7 |
| | 2.1.2. Botanical description of the genus *Myricaria*................... | 7 |
| | 2.1.3. Botanical description of *Myricaria germanica* (L.) Desv......... | 8 |
| | **2.2. CHEMISTRY**................................................................... | 13 |
| | 2.2.1. Chemical constituents of some Tamaricaceous plants........... | 13 |
| | 2.2.2. Chemical constituents of the genus *Myricaria*................... | 13 |
| |     2.2.2.1. *Myricaria bracteata*................................................. | 14 |
| |     2.2.2.2. *Myricaria alopecuroides*........................................... | 15 |
| |     2.2.2.3. *Myricaria elegans*..................................................... | 16 |
| |     2.2.2.4. *Myricaria paniculata*................................................. | 16 |
| |     2.2.2.5. *Myricaria laxiflora*.................................................... | 17 |
| |     2.2.2.6. *Myricaria longifolia*.................................................. | 17 |
| |     2.2.2.7. *Myricaria germanica*................................................ | 17 |
| | **2.3. FOLK MEDICINE**............................................................ | 18 |
| | 2.3.1. Folk medicinal uses of some Tamaricaceous plants............... | 18 |
| | 2.3.2. Folk medicinal uses of the genus *Myricaria*........................ | 19 |
| | 2.3.3. Folk medicinal uses of *Myricaria germanica*....................... | 19 |
| | 2.3.4. *Myricaria germanica* in Tibetan medicine............................ | 20 |
| | **2.4. BIOLOGICAL ACTIVITY**................................................ | 23 |
| | 2.4.1. Biological activities of *Myricaria* species............................. | 23 |
| | 2.4.2. Biological activities of *Myricaria germanica*....................... | 24 |

I

# 3 MATERIALS, APPARATUS AND METHODS .................................... 26

**3.1. Materials**.................................................................................................. 26
3.1.1. Plant materials.................................................................................... 26

**3.2. Phytochemical screening: General tests for preliminary screening of phyto-constituents**........................................................................................ 26
3.2.1. Flavonoids......................................................................................... 26
3.2.2. Coumarins ........................................................................................ 26
3.2.3. Steroids and/ or triterpenoids............................................................ 26
3.2.4. Carbohydrates and / or glycosides.................................................... 26
3.2.5. Saponins............................................................................................ 27
3.2.6. Phenolics........................................................................................... 27
3.2.7. Alkaloids........................................................................................... 27
3.2.8. Anthraquinones................................................................................. 27

**3.3. Phytochemical investigation of *Myricaria germanica* (L) Desv. (Tamaricaceae)**.................................................................................. 28
3.3.1. Plant extract...................................................................................... 28
3.3.2. Authentic reference materials........................................................... 28
3.3.3. Chromatographic materials............................................................... 28
    3.3.3.1. Paper chromatography............................................................. 28
    3.3.3.2. Solvent systems for paper chromatography ........................... 28
    3.3.3.3. Column chromatography ........................................................ 29
    3.3.3.4. Solvent system for column chromatography.......................... 29
    3.3.3.5. Spray reagents and test solutions............................................ 29

**3.4. Materials for biological study**.......................................................... 30
3.4.1. Chemicals and drugs......................................................................... 30
3.4.2. Human tumour cell lines for cytotoxic activity................................ 31

**3.5. Apparatus**............................................................................................ 31
3.5.1. Rotary evaporator ............................................................................ 31
3.5.2. Ultra-Violet lamp ............................................................................. 31

| | |
|---|---|
| 3.5.3. Ultra-Violet spectrophotometer..................................................... | 31 |
| 3.5.4. Open glass columns..................................................................... | 31 |
| 3.5.5. Rectangular glass jars of different size and micro-pipette ............... | 31 |
| 3.5.6. Nuclear Magnetic Resonance....................................................... | 31 |
| 3.5.7. Inverted microscope..................................................................... | 32 |
| 3.5.8. Orbital shaker............................................................................... | 32 |
| 3.5.9. Spectrophotometer ELIZA microplate reader................................ | 32 |
| 3.5.10 High resolution ESI-MS................................................................ | 32 |
| | |
| **3.6. Phytochemical methods** ............................................................... | 32 |
| 3.6.1. Chromatographic methods ........................................................... | 32 |
|    3.6.1.1. Paper chromatographic analysis............................................. | 32 |
|    3.6.1.2. Column chromatographic analysis .......................................... | 32 |
|    3.6.1.3. Thin Layer Chromatography.................................................... | 33 |
|    3.6.1.4. Electrophoretic analysis........................................................... | 33 |
| 3.6.2. Chemical methods | 33 |
|    3.6.2.1. Complete (Normal) acid hydrolysis.......................................... | 33 |
|    3.6.2.2. Mild (Controlled) acid hydrolysis ............................................. | 34 |
|    3.6.2.3. Enzymatic hydrolysis ............................................................... | 34 |
| | |
| **3.7. Physical methods** | 34 |
| 3.7.1. UV analysis ................................................................................... | 34 |
| 3.7.2. $^1H$ and $^{13}C$- NMR analysis ........................................................ | 34 |
| 3.7.3. Mass spectrometric analysis ......................................................... | 34 |
| 3.7.4. Flame atomic absorption analysis ................................................. | 35 |
| 3.7.5. $[\alpha]_D^{27}$ recording ....................................................................... | 35 |
| | |
| **3.8. Methods for the Biological Investigation of the Aqueous Ethanol Extract of *Myricaria germanica*, its column chromatographic fractions and isolated compounds**........................................................................................ | 35 |
| 3.8.1. Cell culture.................................................................................... | 36 |
| 3.8.2. Sulforhodamine B colorimetric assay ............................................ | 37 |
| 3.8.3. Determination of caspase-3 activity .............................................. | 39 |

3.8.4. Analysis of cell cycle distribution .................................................... 42

3.8.5. Determination of Poly (ADP-ribose) polymerase (PARP) enzyme activity ... 44

# 4 PHENOLIC CONSTITUENTS OF AERIAL PARTS OF AQUEOUS ALCOHOL EXTRACT OF *Myricaria germanica* (l.) Desv.: RESULTS AND DISCUSSION.................................................................. 46

4.1. Phytochemical screening of the aerial parts of *Myricaria germanica*............ 46

4.2. Extraction.......................................................................................... 46

    4.2.1. Qualitative phenolic analysis of the extract........................................ 46

    4.2.2. Chromatographic investigation......................................................... 47

4.3. Isolation of compounds (1-20) from the column fractions (I- XII) ............... 50

4.4. Paper chromatographic analysis of fractions (I- XII) .............................. 50

**Fraction I** ............................................................................................ 51

**Fraction I-1**......................................................................................... 51

Isolation of compound **1** ........................................................................ 51

Identification of compound **1**: 3-Methoxygallic acid 5-sodium sulphate ............. 51

**Fraction II** ........................................................................................... 54

Isolation of compound **2** ........................................................................ 54

Identification of compound **2: New natural product, Kaempferide 3, 7-disodium sulphate**.............................................................................................. 54

**Fraction III**.......................................................................................... 60

Isolation of compounds **3** and **4**.............................................................. 60

Identification of compound **3**: Kaempferide 3-sodium sulphate......................... 60

Identification of compound **4**: Tamarexitin 3- sodium sulphate ....................... 63

**Fraction IV**.......................................................................................... 66

Isolation of compounds **5** and **6** ............................................................. 66

Identification of compound **5**: Gallic acid ................................................... 66

Identification of compound **6**: 3-Methoxygallic acid....................................... 69

| | |
|---|---:|
| **Fraction V**.................................................................................................. | 72 |
| Isolation of compound **7**.................................................................................. | 72 |
| Identification of compound **7**: 2, 3-di-*O*- Galloyl-(α/β)-glucose ........................ | 72 |
| | |
| **Fraction VI**................................................................................................. | 76 |
| Isolation of compounds **8, 9** and **10**................................................................ | 76 |
| Identification of compound **8**: Quercetin 3-*O*-β-glucuronide............................. | 76 |
| Identification of compound **9**: Kaempferol 3-*O*-β-glucuronide .......................... | 79 |
| Identification of compound **10**: **New natural product, Tamarixetin 3-*O*-β-glucuronide**................................................................................................ | 82 |
| | |
| **Fraction VII**................................................................................................ | 87 |
| Isolation of compound **11** and **12**..................................................................... | 87 |
| Identification of compound **11**: 1, 3-di-*O*-Galloyl-β-glucose............................ | 87 |
| Identification of compound **12**: **New natural product, 2, 4-di-*O*-Galloyl (α/β) glucopyranose**............................................................................................ | 92 |
| | |
| **Fraction VIII** ............................................................................................. | 98 |
| Isolation of compound **13**................................................................................ | 98 |
| Identification of compound **13**: 2, 6-di-*O*- Galloyl-(α/β)-glucose...................... | 98 |
| | |
| **Fraction IX** ................................................................................................ | 105 |
| Isolation of compound **14** ............................................................................... | 105 |
| Identification of compound **14**: Tamarixellagic acid......................................... | 105 |
| | |
| **Fraction X** .................................................................................................. | 117 |
| Isolation of compounds **15** and **16**................................................................... | 117 |
| Identification of compound **15**: Kaempferol 3-*O*-α-rhamnopyranoside................ | 117 |
| Identification of compound **16**: Quercetin 3-*O*-α-rhamnopyranoside.................. | 122 |

| | |
|---|---|
| **Fraction XI** | 126 |
| Isolation of compounds **17, 17\*, 18** and **19** | 126 |
| Identification of compound **17**: Kaempferol | 126 |
| Identification of compound **17\***: Kaempferide | 129 |
| Identification of compound **18**: Tamarixetin | 131 |
| Identification of compound **19**: Quercetin | 134 |
| | |
| **Fraction XII** | 136 |
| Isolation of compound **20** | 136 |
| Identification of compound **20: New natural product, *N-trans*-3-hydroxy 4-methoxy cinnamoyltyramine (Tamgermanetin)** | 136 |

## 5 BIOLOGICAL INVESTIGATION OF *Myricaria germanica* (L.) Desv. AERIAL PARTS EXTRACT, COULMN FRACTIONS AND ISOLATED COMPOUNDS: RESULTS AND DISCUSSION .......................................... 144

| | |
|---|---|
| 5.1. Cytotoxicity assessment | 144 |
| 5.2. Assessment of cell cycle distribution | 146 |
| 5.3. Assessment of PARP and caspase-3 enzyme activity | 149 |
| Conclusion | 150 |
| Recommendations | 153 |
| | |
| SUMMARY | 155 |
| REFERENCES | 164 |
| APPENDIX | 178 |

## LIST OF TABLES

| No. | | Page |
|---|---|---|
| 1. | Examples of traditional plant derived medicines............................................. | 4 |
| 2. | Solvent systems for paper chromatography................................................. | 28 |
| 3. | Phytochemical screening of the aerial parts of *Myricaria germanica*............ | 46 |
| 4. | Qualitative phenolic analysis of extract......................................................... | 47 |
| 5. | Characteristics of the column fractions (I– XII) of the extract.................. | 49 |
| 6. | Chromatographic and spectral data of compound (**1**)................................... | 52 |
| 7. | Chromatographic and spectral data of compounds (**2, 2a, 2b**)..................... | 56 |
| 8. | Chromatographic and spectral data of compound (**3**) ................................. | 61 |
| 9. | Chromatographic and spectral data of compound (**4**) ................................. | 64 |
| 10. | Chromatographic and spectral data of compound (**5**) ................................. | 67 |
| 11. | Chromatographic and spectral data of compound (**6**).................................. | 70 |
| 12. | Chromatographic and spectral data of compound (**7**) ................................. | 73 |
| 13. | Chromatographic and spectral data of compound (**8**) ................................. | 77 |
| 14. | Chromatographic and spectral data of compound (**9**)................................... | 80 |
| 15. | Chromatographic and spectral data of compound (**10** and **10a**) ................. | 83 |
| 16. | Chromatographic and spectral data of compound (**11**)................................ | 89 |
| 17. | Chromatographic and spectral data of compound (**12** and **12a**).................. | 94 |
| 18. | Chromatographic and spectral data of compound (**13** and **13a**)................. | 100 |
| 19. | Chromatographic and spectral data of compound (**14**) and its hydrolysates...................................................................................................... | 109 |
| 20. | Chromatographic and spectral data of compound (**15**)................................ | 118 |
| 21. | Chromatographic and spectral data of compound (**16**)................................ | 123 |
| 22. | Chromatographic and spectral data of compound (**17**)................................ | 127 |
| 23. | Chromatographic and spectral data of compound (**17∗**) ............................. | 129 |
| 24. | Chromatographic and spectral data of compound (**18**)................................ | 132 |
| 25. | Chromatographic and spectral data of compound (**19**)................................ | 134 |
| 26. | Chromatographic and spectral data of compound (**20**)................................ | 138 |
| 27. | Cytotoxicity parameters of the crude extract, column fractions and isolated compounds against different solid tumor cell lines................................ | 145 |

## LIST OF FIGURES

1. *Myricaria germanica* (L.) Desv. Distribution in Europe........................... 11
2. German tamarisk shrub *(Myricaria germanica)*............... 11
3. German tamarisk branch (*Myricaria germanica*)................................. 12
4. German tamarisk inflorescence (*Myricaria germanica*)........................... 12
5. $^1$H-NMR spectrum of compound (**1**) ................................................. 53
6. $^{13}$C-NMR spectrum of compound (**1**)................................................. 53
7. $^1$H-NMR spectrum of compound (**2**) .................................................. 59
8. $^1$H-NMR spectrum of compound (**3**) ................................................ 62
9. $^1$H-NMR spectrum of compound (**4**) ................................................ 65
10. $^{13}$C-NMR spectrum of compound (**4**) ................................................ 65
11. ESI-MS spectrum of compound (**5**) ................................................. 68
12. $^{13}$C-NMR spectrum of compound (**5**) ................................................ 68
13. Negative ESI-MS of compound (**6**) .................................................... 71
14. $^{13}$C-NMR spectrum of compound (**6**)................................................. 71
15. Negative ESI-MS spectrum of compound (**7**)...................................... 74
16. Negative ESI-MS spectrum of compound (**7a**)...................................... 74
17. $^1$H-NMR spectrum of compound (**7**) .................................................. 75
18. $^{13}$C-NMR spectrum of compound (**7**) .................................................. 75
19. $^1$H-NMR spectrum of compound (**8**).................................................. 78
20. $^{13}$C-NMR spectrum of compound (**8**) ................................................ 78
21. $^1$H-NMR spectrum of compound (**9**)................................................... 81
22. ESI-MS spectrum of compound (**10**)................................................. 85
23. $^1$H –NMR spectrum of compound (**10**)............................................... 85
24. $^{13}$C-NMR spectrum of compound (**10**)............................................... 86
25. ESI-MS spectrum of compound (**11**)................................................. 90
26. $^1$H-NMR spectrum of compound (**11**)........................................ ............ 91

| 27. | $^{13}$C-NMR spectrum of compound (11)............................................... | 91 |
| 28. | ESI-MS spectrum of compound (12)................................................. | 95 |
| 29. | $^{1}$H-NMR spectrum of sugar protons of compound (12)............................ | 96 |
| 30. | $^{1}$H-NMR spectrum of aromatic proton of compound (12)................... ...... | 96 |
| 31. | $^{1}$H- $^{1}$H COSY spectrum of compound (12) ....................................... | 97 |
| 32. | Negative ESI-MS spectrum of compound (13)....................................... | 102 |
| 33. | Negative FAB-MS of compound (13a)................................................ | 102 |
| 34. | $^{1}$H-NMR spectrum of compound (13).................................................. | 103 |
| 35. | $^{1}$H-NMR spectrum of compound (13a)................................................ | 103 |
| 36. | $^{13}$C – NMR spectrum of compound (13)................................................ | 104 |
| 37. | Positive ESI-MS spectrum of 4, 6-$O$-hexahydroxybiphenoyl glucose......... | 112 |
| 38. | Positive ESI-MS spectrum of compound (14)....................................... | 112 |
| 39. | Positive ESI-MS spectrum of compound (14a).................................... | 113 |
| 40. | Negative ESI-MS spectrum of compound (14a)................................... | 113 |
| 41. | $^{1}$H-NMR spectrum of compound (14)............................................... | 114 |
| 42. | $^{1}$H-NMR spectrum of compound (14a)............................................. | 115 |
| 43. | $^{13}$C – NMR spectrum of compound (14)............................................. | 116 |
| 44. | ESI-MS spectrum of compound (15)................................................. | 120 |
| 45. | $^{1}$H-NMR spectrum of compound (15)............................................... | 120 |
| 46. | $^{13}$C-NMR spectrum of compound (15).............................................. | 121 |
| 47. | Negative ESI-MS spectrum of compound (16)..................................... | 124 |
| 48. | $^{1}$H- NMR spectrum of compound (16).............................................. | 125 |
| 49. | $^{13}$C- NMR spectrum of compound (16)............................................. | 125 |
| 50. | ESI -MS spectrum of compound (17)................................................. | 127 |

| | | |
|---|---|---|
| 51. | $^1$H- NMR spectrum of compound (**17**)..................................................... | 128 |
| 52. | $^1$H- NMR spectrum of compound (**17\***)................................................... | 130 |
| 53. | $^{13}$C- NMR spectrum of compound (**17\***)................................................. | 130 |
| 54. | $^1$H- NMR spectrum of compound (**18**)..................................................... | 133 |
| 55. | $^{13}$C- NMR spectrum of compound (**18**)................................................... | 133 |
| 56. | ESI-MS spectrum of compound (**19**)......................................................... | 135 |
| 57. | $^1$H- NMR spectrum of compound (**19**)..................................................... | 135 |
| 58. | Positive ESI-MS of compound (**20**)........................................................... | 140 |
| 59. | Negative ESI-MS of compound (**20**).......................................................... | 140 |
| 60. | $^1$H-NMR spectrum of compound (**20**)...................................................... | 141 |
| 61. | $^{13}$C-NMR spectrum of compound (**20**).................................................... | 141 |
| 62. | $^1$H-$^1$H COSY spectrum of aliphatic protons of compound (**20**)................. | 142 |
| 63. | $^1$H-$^1$H COSY spectrum of aromatic protons of compound (**20**)............... | 143 |
| 64. | Effect of tamarixellagic acid and tamgermanitin on the cell cycle distribution of Huh-7 liver cancer cell lines............................ | 147 |
| 65. | Effect of tamarixellagic acid and tamgermanitin on the cell cycle distribution of MCF-7 breast cancer cell lines.................................................. | 148 |
| 66. | Effect of tamarixellagic acid and tamgermanitin on PARP and caspase-3 enzyme activity............................................................................... | 149 |

## LIST OF ABBREVIATIONS

| | |
|---|---|
| 2DPC | Two dimensional paper chromatography |
| HOAc-6 | 6% acetic acid |
| CoPC | Comparitive Paper Chromatography |
| $^{13}$C-NMR | Carbon-13 Nuclear Magnetic Resonance |
| DMSO-$d_6$ | deutrated dimethylsulfoxide |
| DNA | Deoxyribonucleic acid |
| $^1$H-NMR | Proton Nuclear Magnetic Resonance |
| ax. | axial |
| eq. | equatorial |
| EDTA | Ethylenediaminetetraacetic acid |
| ELISA | Enzyme-linked immunosorbent assay |
| ESI-MS | Electro Spray Ionization Mass Spectrometry |
| IC$_{50}$ | half maximal inhibitory concentration |
| FAB-MS | Fast Atomic Bombardment Mass Spectrometry |
| FBS | Fetal bovine serum |
| Fig. | Figure |
| FTMS | **F**ourier **T**ransform **M**ass **S**pectrometry |
| g | gram |
| HMBC | Heteronuclear Multiple Bond Connectivity |
| HSQC | Heteronuclear Single Quantum Coherence |
| Huh-7 | Human hepatocellular carcinoma cell line |
| Hz | Hertz |
| J value | Coupling constant |
| mM | milliMolar |
| M.wt. | Molecular weight |
| m/z | Mass to charge ratio |
| mg | milligram |
| min. | minute |
| Mr | Molecular wieght |
| MS | Mass Spectrometry |
| MCF-7 | Breast adenocarcinoma cell line |
| nm | nanometer |
| PARP | Poly (ADP-ribose) polymerase |
| PBS | Phospahte Buffered Saline |
| PC-3 | Prostate adenocarcinoma cell line |
| PC | Paper Chromatography |
| PPC | preparative paper chromatography |
| ppm | part per million |
| ppt | precipitate |
| $R_f$ | Retardation factor |
| RNA | Ribonucleic acid |
| RNase | Ribonuclease |
| rpm | revolutions per minute |
| RT | room temperature |
| TCA | trichloroacetic acid |
| TLC | Thin Layer Chromatography |
| UV | Ultraviolet |
| V | Visible |

| | |
|---|---|
| δ | Chemical shift |
| λ | wave length |
| μ | micro |
| μl | microliter |
| $[\alpha]_D^C$ | Specific rotation |
| SRB assay | **Sulfo**rodamine **B** assay |
| cm | Centimeter |
| Diam. | Diameter |
| N.R.C. | National Research Center |
| EtOAC | ethylacetate |
| $CD_3(2)CO$ | deuteroacetone (acetone-$d_6$) |
| CF | Column Fractionation |
| Amm. | ammonia |
| BAW | Butanol:Acetic acid:Water |
| Aq.MeOH | aqueous methanol |

# 1. INTRODUCTION

In several modern countries, the fight for the acceptance and registration of phytopharmaceuticals as drugs was successful. Most of these plant derivatives have been already registered as conventional drug, which mean that they meet the same stringent criteria of quality, efficacy and safety as synthetic drugs. Besides, these criteria have stimulated the search for the active principles in plant extracts, which show potent biological activities. Therefore, search for the active principles became an important prerequisite for the developmental procedures aiming to bring a bioactive plant derivative to the stage of a marketable drug.

Many of the plant derived drugs which are already in use nowadays are rich in phenolic metabolites. Phenolic compounds are ubiquitous in plants which collectively synthesize several thousands of different chemical structures characterized by hydroxylated aromatic ring(s), known as phenols (Haslam, 1996; Hemingway *et al.*, 1999).

Many of the already usable drugs are rich in phenolics, e.g. derivatives of *Crataegus*, *Silybum*, *Urtica*, *Paeonia*, *Camellia*, *Glycine max* and *Echinacea*. In many instances, the used plant derived drugs are actually pure phenolics isolated from terrestrial plants. Simple phenolics show a wide range of antioxidant activities in vitro (Rice-Evans *et al.*, 1995) and are thought to exert protective effects against major diseases such as cancer. Oxidative stress imposed by reactive oxygen species (ROS) indeed plays a crucial role in the pathophysiology associated with neoplasia.

The ROS-induced development of cancer involves for example malignant transformation due to DNA mutations as well as modification of gene expression through epigenetic mechanisms (Lee *et al.*, 2006). A wide range of molecular, *in vitro* epidemiological studies have been undertaken to confirm the postulated effects of these compounds. Epidemiological studies analyse the health implications of phenolic plant extracts and their phenolic isolates on various pathological situations. The specific actions of individual phenols are supported by *in vitro* assays (Brown *et al.*, 2005; Choueiri *et al.*, 2006; Haddad *et al.*, 2006; Szaever *et al.*, 2006).

Advances in the field of polyphenolics (tannins), particularly hydrolysable tannins, have remarkably changed the concept of tannins. The name "tannin" no longer means a mixture of unidentified compounds, but refers to each individual compound in the tannin family and also to the whole family in a similar fashion to other natural organic compounds such as alkaloids and terpenoids. Phenolics and their glycosides have therefore, received during the last few decades, an increasing attention from chemists and pharmacologists. Interest on the part of chemists has been twofold: natural product chemists have propped terrestrial plants as sources of new unusual phenolics and other organic molecules, while synthetic chemists have followed by targeting these novel structures for developments of new analogues and new synthetic methodologies and strategies. Interest on the part of pharmacologists has focused on their potential applications for treating human diseases.

Plant phenols, including polyphenols are among the most potent and therapeutically promising bioactive substances. Previous comprehensive studies proved that plant phenols possess diverse effects on biological systems. The diversity of their structures is the basis of the recent increase in the detection of the various biological and pharmacological activities which have been extensively researched such as antitumor, antibacterial, enzyme inhibitory, antihepatotoxic, antioxidant, antiallergic, anti-inflammatory, antiosteoporotic, analgesic, antiviral and immunomodulating (Akagawa and Suyama, 2001; Germano *et al.*, 2005; Haslam, 1996; Lee *et al.*, 2005; Wang *et al.*, 1999).

It should be also noted that a remarkable number of the traditional plant-derived medicines are extracts rich in phenolics (Anne, 2000; Brown, 1999; Brynin, 2002; Haslam *et al.*, 1989; Morazzoni and Bombvardelli, 1996). (Table 1)

Polyphenolic compounds are well known to exhibit antioxidant properties (Bouchet *et al.*, 1998) and can also act as a direct scavenger molecules (Hagimasi *et al.*, 2000). They can prevent lipid peroxidation and biological damage caused by free radicals formed under oxidative stress.

The confirmed antibiotic activity of phenolics in a human body was suggested to result from direct interaction of these plant metabolites with microbes, as concluded from established polyphenol toxicity towards microorganisms in a number of biological experiments (Nitta *et al.*, 2002).

It is proved that such interaction, i.e. inhibition of pathogenic bacteria and inactivation of their produced toxins, occurs in the digestive tract, thus providing a rational but simplified explanation for beneficial effects in gastro-intestinal upsets such as diarrhea. The potential of antibacterial and antiviral activities of tannins therefore, depends on their structures (Fukushi *et al.*, 1989).

Many dimeric ellagitannins also were found to inhibit replication of human immunodeficiency virus (HIV). It was proved that the antiviral activity of these ellagitannins may be ascribable to the inhibition of adsorption of HIV on the cells, and also to other effect such as inhibition of reverse transcriptase activity (Asanaka *et al.*, 1988; Swain *et al.*, 1977).

## Table (1): Examples of traditional plant derived medicines rich in phenolics:

| Common Name | Latin Name | Part Used | Active Ingredients | Main Medicinal Activity |
|---|---|---|---|---|
| Tree peony | *Paeonia lactiflora* | Outer skin of the roots | Gallotannin | Cure disorder of the blood stream including high blood pressure |
| Hawthorn | *Crataegus laevigata* | Leaves & flowers | Flavonoids & oligomeric proanthocyanidins | Treatment of cardiovascular diseases |
| Billberry | *Vaccinium myrtillus* | Fruits | Anthocyanins | Improve visual function |
| Green tea | *Camellia sinensis* | Leaves | Catechins | Antioxidant & antibacterial |
| Grape seed | *Vitis species* | Seeds | Proanthocyandins | Antioxidant |
| Soyabean | *Glycine max* | Hypocotyls | Isoflavones | Estrogen like action & alleviate menopausal disorders |
| Ginkgo biloba | *Ginkgo biloba* | Leaves | Flavonol glycosides | Cure disorders of central nervous system & blood vessels |
| Purple cone flower | *Echinacea purpurea* | Shoots & roots | Phenolic acids derivatives | Immunostimulant & respiratory infections |

Due to the remarkable situation of many natural phenolics as plant derived drugs and to the fact that the constitutive phenolics of many of the wild plants have not been subjected to comprehensive biological and chemical investigations, one can therefore come to the conclusion that the discovery of bioactive phenolics derived from these plants would merit high attention.

On the other hand, the most common tumors of the adult are resistant to available antineoplastic drugs (Sheet, 1996; Thornes and O' Kennedy, 1997) and the majority of these agents have only limited anti-solid tumor activity. Natural products, including plant phenolics provide a major source of chemical diversity that has consistently proven its value for the development of novel drugs for more effective antineoplastic agents. Nature provides candidate compounds which have more "drug-like" properties (i.e., in terms of absorption and metabolism) as well as a greater chemical diversity (i.e., to allow for structure-activity studies), (Harvey, 1999). In an *in vitro* survey of preventive agents against tumor promotion from medicinal plants, polyphenols such as (-)-epigallocatechin gallate (EGCG) (Yoshizawa *et al.*, 1987) and pentagalloylglucose, pedunculagin and chebulinic acid etc. were found to possess promising anti-cancer activity, e.g. they exhibit a competitive binding activity to TPA receptor in a particulate fraction of mouse skin (Yoshizawa *et al.*, 1992).

On the basis of the above given criteria, the present study will investigate the cytotoxicity and the constitutive phenolics of *Myricaria germanica* DESV aiming to achieve candidate phenolics which could be used for the development of effective antineoplastic agents.

The genus *Myricaria* belongs to the family Tamaricaceae, which comprises four genera and about 110 species widely distributed in Europe, Africa, and Asia (Qaiser and Perveen, 2004). Many of these species grow on saline soils, tolerating up to 15,000-ppm soluble salt and can also tolerate alkaline conditions. In view of this fact, the capability of these plants on synthesizing and accumulating sulphate conjugates of flavonols, phenyl propanoids and other phenolics (Nawwar *et al.*, 1976; Souleman *et al.*, 1998) is thus not all that surprising. Among the ten *Myricaria* species, *Myricaria germanica* (L.) Desv, known in English as German false tamarisk or German tamarisk is growing in temperate regions. The plant is a folk medicinal plant whose bark extract has been used in folk medicine for treatment of jaundice, while the infusion of the leaves was used as analgesic and was found to possess antimicrobial activity and the ability to control chronic bronchitis (Kirbag *et al.*, 2009; Phani *et al.*, 2009). The only previous phytochemical investigation of the plant leaf cuticular waxes has led to the isolation and characterization of a number of long-chain alkanediols (Jetter, 2000). As long as the available literature is concerned this plant has not been subjected to any previous phytochemical investigation of its constitutive phenolics except one article descrbing the isolation of some flavonoids written in Chinese (La *et al.*, 2011). Due to our interest in the chemistry and biology of the phenolic constituents in Tamaricaceae (Nawwar *et al.*, 1982; Nawwar *et al.*, 1984; Nawwar *et al.*, 1994a; Nawwar and Hussein, 1994b). In the present work, we investigated in- depth the phenolic constituents in *Myricaia germanica*, as well as, cytotoxic effect against three different solid tumor cell lines, namely liver (Huh-7), breast (MCF-7), and prostate (PC-3).

## Aim of work:

- Isolation of phenolic compounds from the aqueous ethanol aerial parts extract of *Myricaria germanica* DESV.

- Identification of the isolated phenolics using chemical analysis, conventional, advanced spectroscopic and spectrometric techniques.

- Investigation of the extract, its chromatographic fractions and the isolated pure compounds for cytotoxicity against three different solid tumor cell lines, namely liver (Huh-7), breast (MCF-7) and prostate (PC-3).

## 2. REVIEW OF LITERATURE

### 2.1. BOTANY

#### 2.1.1. Botanical description of the family Tamaricaceae:

Tamaricaceae is a small family of 4 genera and 110 species (Mabberley, 1987), temperate in distribution, usually in sandy tracts and maritime deserts of Europe, Asia and Africa (Qaiser, 1982).

In addition, the family members are capable of accumulating salt in special glands in its leaves, and then excrete it onto the leaf surface. Foliage of salt cedar is often covered with a bloom of salt (Decker, 1961; Mozingo, 1987). These salts accumulate in the surface layer of soil when plants drop their leaves (Mozingo, 1987).

Tamaricaceous plants are shrubs, subshrubs, or trees. **Leaves:** alternate, exstipulate, usually sessile, small, and scale-like, herbaceous or fleshy, mostly with salt secreting glands, persistent; **inflorescence:** simple racemes, panicles or spikes (*Tamarisceae*); **flowers:** bisexual, actinomorphic, 4-5 merous; sepals and petals free or connate at the base; anthers 2-celled, obtuse or apiculate, dehiscing by longitudinal slit; pollen grains tricolpate, with smooth wall; ovary superior, 1-locular; placentas 3-5, arising from the base; carpels 2-5, with parietal placenta; ovules usually numerous, anatropous; styles as many as the carpels, short, usually 2-5, free, sometimes united; stigmas capitates, sometimes sessile; fruit capsule, 3-5 angled, pyramidal, dehiscing by 3-5 valves from apex to the base ; **seeds:** many, hairy all around or with a tuft of hairs; endosperm absent (*Tamarisceae*) with straight embryo and flat cotyledons (Boulos, 1999; Qaiser, 1982; Yang and Gaskin, 2007)

#### 2.1.2. Botanical description of the genus *Myricaria*:

*Myricaria* comprises about ten species in Europe, Africa and Asia; four of them are endemic in China. Many of these species grow on saline soils, tolerating up to 15,000-ppm soluble salt and can tolerate alkaline conditions (Qaiser and Perveen, 2004).

*Myricaria* Desvaux: shrubs, rarely subshrubs, deciduous, erect or prostrate. **Leaves:** simple, alternate, sessile, usually densely arranged on green young branches of current year and margin entire. **Flowers:** are bisexual, shortly petiolate, clustered into terminal or lateral racemes or panicles; bracts broadly or narrowly membranous along margin. Calyx 5-fid; lobes often membranous along margin. Petals 5, pink, white, or purplish red, obovate, narrowly elliptic, or obovate-oblong, apex obtuse or emarginate, often incurved, usually persistent in fruit. Stamens 10: 5 long and 5 short; filaments ca. 1/2 or 2/3 united, rarely free; anthers 2-thecate, longitudinally dehiscent, yellow. Pistils consisting of 3 carpels; ovary 3-angled; placentation basal; ovules numerous; stigmas capitate, 3-lobed. Capsule 3-septicidal. Seeds numerous, apex awned; awns white villous throughout or on more than half; endosperm absent(Qaiser, 1976a).

### 2.1.3. Botanical description of *Myricaria germanica* (L.) Desv

Among *Myricaria* species, *Myricaria germanica* (L.) Desv., known in English as German false tamarisk or German tamarisk is growing in temperate regions especially in the Mediterranean area. It is the only species of its family Tamaricaceae in Central Europe (Schönefelder and Bresinsky, 1990). It is nearly allied to *Tamarix* plants, but it differs in having ten stamens to each flower. The branches are erect, rather sturdier than in the true *Tamarix*, the leaves are pale glaucous hue and the flowers are white or rosy in June (Pengyun and Yaojia 1990).

*Myricaria germanica* (German tamarisk) is up to 2 m tall evergreen shrub (Fig. 2). Very small, oblong to lanceolate shaped, opposite **leaves** sit on their upright, rod-like branches (2-5 mm long, scale-like, overlapping often tile-shaped) that are pressed against the younger branches, extending to older however more the leaves are colored gray-green (Fig. 3). **The inflorescences** are terminal, especially on the main branches, and form simple or paniculate branched, compact bunches (Fig. 4). The inconspicuous individual **flowers** consist of 5 (rarely 4) lineal sepals (3 mm long) and 5 (rarely 4) white to light pink. The 10 anthers are purple or red, 5 stamens are about as long as the calyx, 5 little longer In good weather, the flowers are pollinated by insects that are attracted by nectar. In rainy weather, when the flowers remain closed until half full, it can also cause self-pollination Flowering season is from May to August, but it is by the location (especially the sea level) influenced. The 12 mm long gray-green capsules are narrow pyramidal, narrow and often crowded reddish. The brown **seeds** weigh only 0,065 mg, they are a 5 to 7 mm long spring-like head of hair (pappus ) equipped and can be described as typical screen plane. Strong root system of German tamarisk contributes to strengthening the ground in their habitat. In specifying the maximum age, the authors disagree: There are between 10 and 70 years specified (Bachmann, 1997; Frisendahl, 1921).

The scope of re-introduction as a measure for plant species protection is increasing, but as long as no standardized methods are available, species-specific assessments are necessary to determine whether seeds, adult plants or plant fragments should be used. The endangered German False Tamarisk (*Myricaria germanica*), which occurs on gravel bars along pre-alpine rivers, is difficult to grow from seeds. Thus, propagation of stem cuttings was investigated as an alternative method. Experiments were conducted in a greenhouse and a field site with three treatments: cutting length 5 or 10 cm, vertical burial 5 or 10 cm, and water level low or high. Plants grown in the greenhouse were transplanted to the River Isar to test establishment of rooted cuttings on gravel bars. The cuttings in the greenhouse showed high survival (34-96 %). Survival and biomass production were greatest for 10-cm cuttings buried at 10-cm depth, while only one of the 5-cm cuttings survived at this depth, and no significant effect of variation in water level was observed. None of the cuttings transplanted to field sites survived, most likely because of drought stress and competition. We conclude that for re-introduction of *Myricaria germanica* rooted cuttings can be easily produced in large quantities, while transplantation to near-natural environments has to be improved to reduce mortality (Christiane and Johannes, 2012).

It should be mentioned, that some articles in literature are focusing on molecular phylogency of *Myricaria* and their taxonomy (Chen, 2013; Wang *et al.*, 2009)

## Distribution of *Myricaria germanica* (L) Desv.

The German tamarisk occurs in the European mountains, Asia Minor, Armenia, the Caucasus, Iran, and Afghanistan In Europe (Fig. 1), the range extends from the Pyrenees, to Scandinavia and the Caspian Sea. The southern border is formed by the Pyrenees and the central Apennines, to the Illyrian mountains on the eastern shore of the Adriatic Sea. The type is restricted to the middle and upper reaches of rivers in montane to subalpine regions up to 2350 m. (Hegi, 1975) In the Himalayas there are deposits up to an altitude of 3,950 m.

In the South Island (Canterbury Plains), it was first detected in 1986, where it is understood in some rivers in the propagation. (Sykes and Williams, 1999)

**Habitat:** bank, dry, gravel, hill, margin, moist, mountain, open, riverbed, sand, slope, stone, and track.

## Synonyms of *Myricaria germanica* (L.) Desv.

*English:* False tamarisk, German tamarisk.

German: Rispelstrauch, Deutsche Tamariske.

Botanical synonym: *Tamarix germanica.*

## Taxonomical classification of *Myricaria germanica* (L.) Desv.

- Kingdom: Plantae – Plants
- Subkingdom: Tracheobionta – Vascular plants
- Superdivision: Spermatophyta – Seed plants
- Division: Magnoliophyta – Flowering plants
- Class: Magnoliopsida – Dicotyledons
- Subclass: Dilleniidae
- Order: Violales
- Family: Tamaricaceae – Tamarix family
- Genus: *Myricaria*
- Species: *germanica*

Scientific name: *Myricaria germanica* (L.) Desv.

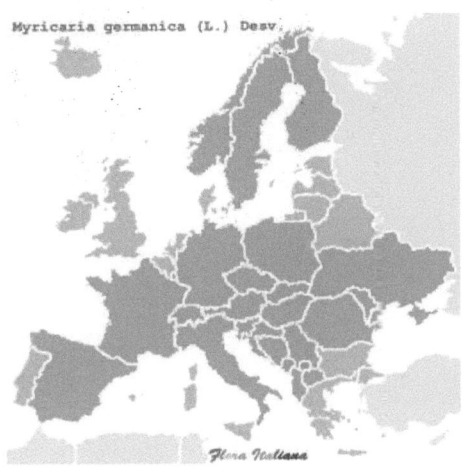

Fig. (1): *Myricaria germanica* (L.) Desv. distribution in Europe

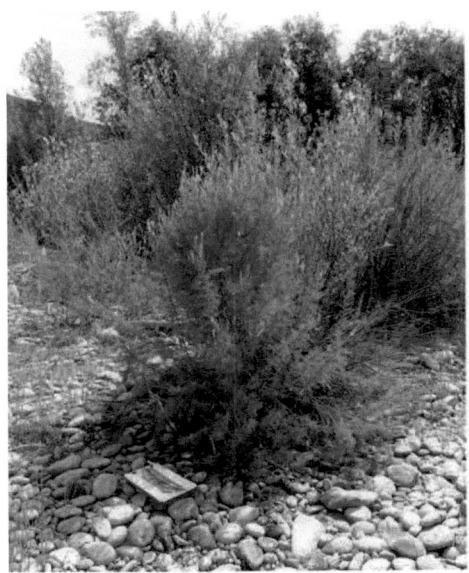

Fig. (2): German tamarisk shrub German tamarisk *(Myricaria germanica)*

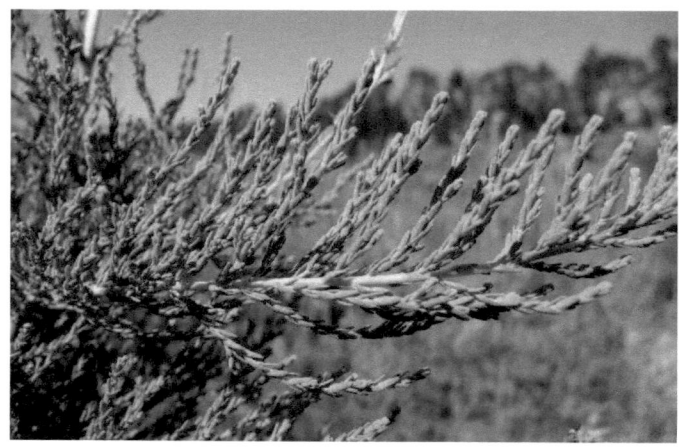

Fig. (3): German tamarisk branch (*Myricaria germanica*)

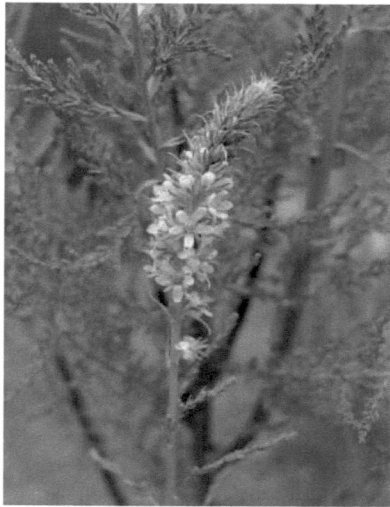

Fig. (4): German tamarisk inflorescence (*Myricaria germanica*)

## 2.2. CHEMISTRY

### 2.2.1. Chemical constituents of some Tamaricaceous plants

Interest in the ellagitannin constituents of medicinal plants has grown in the past decade as a result of their vast structural diversity. They show marked antiviral, antimicrobial, immunomodulatory, antitumor, and hepatic protective activities, which are largely dependent on the phenolic structures (Feldman, 2005; Miyamoto *et al.*, 1993a; Okuda *et al.*, 1989; Yoshida *et al.*, 2000; Yoshida *et al.*, 2009). Among the different ellagitannin classes, those isolated from tamaricaceous plants which have been described as widely varying in structure, including variations in the type of joining moiety and in the mode of attachment between sugar cores in dimeric and oligomeric structures (Ahemad *et al.*, 1994; Yoshida *et al.*, 1991a; Yoshida *et al.*, 1993a; Yoshida *et al.*, 1993b; Yoshida *et al.*, 1991b). The oligomeric hydrolysable tannins are biogenetically the products of intermolecular oxidative C-O or C-C coupling among two or more monomeric hydrolysable tannins, and diversity of their structures and wide distribution in various plant families have been revealed by extensive studies during the last decade (Okuda *et al.*, 1990).

### 2.2.2. Chemical constituents of the genus *Myricaria*

Most of the plants from the genus *Myricaria* were found to contain phenolic compounds. It is known that polyphenol natural products are a major group of compounds with widespread distribution and a broad pharmacological profile (Jing *et al.*, 2002; Sticher *et al.*, 1982). Flavonoids are the major and active constituents of the genus *Myricaria* (Quirino and Terabe, 1998).

Several references have been published on the studies of chemical constituents of genus *Myricaria*. Reviews of literature of some of the species of *Myricaria* have been briefly reproduced.

### 2.2.2.1. *Myricaria bracteata*

A capillary zone electrophoresis (CZE) method for determination of six active components from *M. bracteata* Royle and *M. wardii* Marguandts was developed for the first time. The analytes were completely separated within 15 min. The electrophoresis buffer was 25 mmol L-1 sodium borate concentrations. 15% (vol./vol.) acetonitrile (pH 10.20). The correlation coefficient of the calibration curves for the 6 analytes were 0.9998 or 0.9999 over the concentration ranges examined. Recoveries of the 6 constituents ranged from 96.3 to 106.8%. The method, combined with a relatively simple extraction procedure, was successfully used for analysis of these two *Myricaria* species and the assay results were satisfactory. The compounds were identified as 3,4-dimethoxygallicacid, gallic acetate, 7-methoxyquercetin, kaemferol-3-*O*-rhamnoside, 3-dehydroxy-7-acetylquercetin, and gallic acid (Zhao *et al.*, 2005b).

Sixteen compounds were isolated from the ethyl acetate portion of the 95% ethanol extract of *M. bracteata*, and identified as myricarin (1), myricarin B (2), 3 α-hydroxytaraxer-14-en-28-oic acid (3), myricadiol (4), *trans*-ferulic acid 22-hydroxydocosanoic acid ester (5), docosyl-3, 4-dihydroxy-*trans*-cinnamate (6), dillenetin, 3, 5, 4'-trihydroxy-7-methoxyflavone (7), 3, 5, 4'-trihydroxy-7 (8), 3'-dimethoxyflavone, methyl 3 (9), 5-dihydroxy-4-methoxybenzoate (10), 3-hydroxy-4-methoxy cinnamic acid (11), sinapaldehyde (12), vanillin (13), syringaldehyde (14), 3, 3', 4'-trimethoxyellagic acid (15), methyl *p*-hyroxybenzoate (16). Compounds 5, 6, 12-16 were isolated from the genus *Myricaria* for the first time, all of the compounds were isolated from this species for the first time, except for 8 and 9 (Zhang *et al.*, 2011b).

Eleven compounds were isolated from *M. bracteata* and identified as rhamnetin, 3,5,4'-trihydroxy-7,3'-dimethoxyflavone, 3,5,4'-trihydroxy-7-methoxyflavone, quercetin-3-*O*-α-L-rhamnopyranoside, kaempferol, quercetin, chrysoeriol, gallic acid, gallic acid ethylester, β-sitosterol, daucosterol (Zhou *et al.*, 2006).

### 2.2.2.2. *Myricaria alopecuroides*

Biological activity guided purification of the ethylacetate fraction of *M. alopecuroides* yielded eighteen phenolic compounds. Their molecular structures were elucidated by UV, $^1$H, $^{13}$C NMR and MS analysis as quercetin, kaempferol, herbacetin-8-*O*-xylopyranoside, gossypetin-8-*O*-xylopyranoside, myricetin-3-*O*-α-L-arabinofuranoside, quercetin-3-*O*-α-Larabinofuranoside, quercetin-3-*O*-α-L-arabinopyranoside, quercetin-3-*O*-β-L-galactopyranoside, quercetin-3-*O*-(6''-galloyl)-β-L-galactopyranoside, quercetin-5-*O*-α-L-arabinopyranoside, kaempferol-5-*O*-β-D-glucopyranoside, kaempferol-3-*O*-α-L-rhamnopyranoside, kaempferol- 3-*O*-β-D-(6''-p-coumaroyl)-glucopyranoside, apigenin-7-*O*-β-D-(6''-p-coumaroyl)-glucopyranoside, 5-hydroxy-4'-methoxyisoflavone-7-O-β-glucopyranoside, gallic acid, 6-*O*-galloylarbutin and ethylgallate, respectively.(Gendaram *et al.*, 2008).

Investigation of the chemical constituents in the leaves and branches of *M. alopecuroides* using solvent extraction method was employed to extraction and partition. The chemical constituents were isolated by column chromatography on silica gel, Sephadex LH-20, highly porous resin HP-20. The structures of the compounds were elucidated based on physiochemical properties and spectral analysis. Eleven compounds were isolated from this plant and identified as ellagic acid 3,3',4-trimethylether (1), ellagic acid 3,3'-dimethylether (2), isorhamnetin (3), Kaempferol (4), 3, 5-dihydroxy-4-methoxybenzoic acid (5), daucosterol (6), 6,7,10-trihydroxy-8-octadecenoic acid (7), Quercetin (8), gallic acid (9), palmitic acid (10), hexadecanoic acid, 2,3-dihydroxypropyl ester (11). Except 8 and 9, all compounds were isolated from *M. alopecuroides* for the first time. Compound 1, 2, 5, 7, 10, 11 were obtained from the genus Myricaria for the frist time (Li *et al.*, 2010).

An aqueous acetone extract of stems of *M. alopecuroides*, sampled during the flowering period, yielded a new compd. [$C_{27}H_{20}O_{18}$.$2H_2O$; m.p. 230°; [a]D + 48.6° (c 0.5; MeOH)] identified as 1,2,3-dehydrotrigalloyl-α-D-glucose, and given the name myrinin (Chumbalcv *et al.*, 1979).

Two components were isolated from acid hydrolysates of non-fractionated gallotannins of *M. alopecuroides*, dehydrodigallic acid and dehydrotrigallic acid (Chumbalov *et al.*, 1976).

Chromatography on silica gel and thin-layer chromatography on silufol were used to study the ether and EtOAc extracts from *M. alopecuroides*. The methods yielded three compounds, identified as rhamnazin, rhamnetin, and quercetin (Chumbalov *et al.*, 1975).

Gallic acid, the methyl ester of I and 3-methoxy-4, 5-dihydroxybenzoic acid methyl ester were isolated from *M. alopecuroides* (Chumbalov *et al.*, 1974).

### 2.2.2.3. *Myricaria elegans*

The phytochemical screening of *M. elegans* Royle (Tamaricaceae) gave strongly positive results for terpenes. A total of six triterpenes were isolated from the $CHCl_3$ fraction, including eleganene-A, eleganene-B, corsolic acid, betulin, ursolic acid, and erythrodiol (Khan *et al.*, 2010).

Two pentacyclic triterpenes eleganene-A and eleganene-B, along with four known pentacyclic triterpenes betulin, ursolic acid, erythrodiol and corosolic acid were isolated from the aerial parts of *M. elegans* (Ahmad *et al.*, 2008).

### 2.2.2.4. *Myricaria paniculata*

The chemical constituents of *M. paniculata* were isolated in silica gel column chromatography and the structures were elucidated by spectral analysis. Four compounds were isolated from the petroleum ether soluble portion, identified as 28-aldehyde-taraxerenone, 28-hydroxy-taraxerenone, epi-friedelanol, 4-methyl stigmast-7-en-3-ol . Three compounds were isolated from the EtOAc soluble portion, identified as morelloflavone, methyl 3, 5-dihydroxy-4-methoxybenzoate, and 3-hydroxy-4-methoxy cinnamic acid. All of these compounds were isolated from the genus for the first time (Li *et al.*, 2007).

Two new pentacyclic triterpenoids myricarin A and B have been isolated from the stems of *M. paniculata*, together with seven known compounds, myriconal, 28-hydroxy-14-taraxeren-3-one, epi-friedelanol, beta-sitosterol, 4-methyl stigmast-7-en-3-ol, 12-hentriacontanol and 1-triacontanol (Li *et al.*, 2005).

### 2.2.2.5. *Myricaria Laxiflora*

Gallicin is a gallic acid derivative named methyl 3-hydroxy-4,5-dimethoxybenzoate isolated from *M. Laxiflora*.(Wei *et al.*, 2012).

### 2.2.2.6. *Myricaria longifolia*

Aqueous extract of *M. longifolia* was analyzed by HPLC-UV-DAD and LC-MS$^n$. Ellagic acid, gallic acid, rhamnetin, and rutin were identified by comparison to reference substances. In addition, MS revealed the presence of various sulphates of rhamnetin, isorhamnetin, and quercetin. (Obmann *et al.*, 2010).

### 2.2.2.7. *Myricaria germanica*:

Eleven flavonoids were isolated from the 60% acetone ext. of the air-dry twigs of *M. germanica* (Tamaricaceae) which is a kind of famous Tibetan medicine. Their structures were elucidated by spectroscopic analysis and identified as 3,5,4'-trihydroxy-7,3'-dimethoxyflavone (1), 3,5,4'-trihydroxy-7-methoxyflavone (2), rhamnetin (3), 3,5,7-trihydroxy-4'-methoxyflavone (4), tamarixetin (5), kaempferol (6), quercetin-3-$O$-β-D-glucoside (7), kaempferol-3-$O$-β-D-glucuronic acid (8), quercetin-3-$O$-β-D-glucuronic acid (9), quercetrin (10) and afzelin(11), respectively. All compounds. were obtained from *M.germanica* for the first time, and compounds. 4, 5 and 7-11 were obtained from the genus *Myricaria* for the first time (La *et al.*, 2011).

In the leaf, cuticular waxes of *M. germanica* L. four different series of alkanediols were identified: (1) hentriacontanediol isomers with one functional group in the 12-position and a second group in positions ranging from 2 to 18, (2) $C_{30}$-$C_{34}$ alkanediols carrying one hydroxyl function on a primary and one on a secondary carbon atom. (3) homologous series of $C_{25}$-$C_{43}$ beta-diols predominantly with 8,10- and 10,12-functionalities, and (4) homologous series of $C_{39}$-$C_{43}$ *gamma*-diols with a predominance of 8,11- and 10,13-isomers. Primary/secondary diols and *gamma*-diols constituted only trace portions of the total wax mixture. The hentriacontanediols and the beta-diols amounted to 3.5 and 0.6 microg per cm2 of leaf surface area, corresponding to 9 and 2% of the wax mixture, respectively. Based on the different homolog and isomer patterns of respective diol fractions, two independent biosynthetic routes leading to the hentriacontanediols and the beta-diols are proposed (Jetter, 2000).

## 2.3. FOLK MEDICINE

### 2.3.1. Folk medicinal uses of some Tamaricaceous plants:

Some Tamaricaceous plants have been used in folk medicines for various treatment of diseases in East and South east Asia (Parkin *et al.*, 1999), they are used mainly as as anti-inflammatory, antiseptic and anti-pyretic agents (Boulos, 1983). Some species of *Tamarix* and *Myricaria* are cultivated as ornamental plants (Baily, 1950; Lawrence, 1951) and a few are used for afforestationn (Hawkins, 1958; Herriot, 1942). *Tamarix* species are highly adaptable on sandy soils, especially on the sea shore and are extensively employed in these situations as shelter belt plants (Qaiser, 1976b).

In traditional Egyptian medicine, *Tamarix* extracts have been used especially as antiseptic agents. They are also used for tanning and dyeing purposes (El-Sissi *et al.*, 1973; El Ansari *et al.*, 1976). A strong infusion prepared from the galls of *Tamarix gallica* is used in a local application to foul sloughing ulcers and buboes. The powdered galls, which are rich in tannin, form an efficacious ointment in ulcerating piles and anal fissures (Nadkarni, 1976). Also, *Tamarix gallica* leaves and flowers infusion have anti-inflammatory and anti diarrheic proprieties (Ksouri *et al.*, 2009). Leaves decoction and young branches of *Tamarix aphylla* used for oedema of spleen, same decoction mixed with ginger for uterus affections. Bark of large branches, boiled in water with vinegar, is used as lotion against lice. Infusion of galls, used for enteritis and gastralgia (Boulos, 1983). The wood of *Tamarix aphylla* is used in North Arabia and N. Africa for making house raftors. In North Africa, Arabia and Iran, galls called "Takut or Teggant", derived from this species are used for obtaining tannin, used for fine qualities of goat and sheep skins which take up purplish or pink colour (Hutchinson, 1967).

In traditional Chinese medicine, a decoction of *Tamarix chinensis* (known as Chinese Tamarisk extract) is used as a topical application in measles and skin allergies (Perry and Metzger, 1980). *Tamarix pakistanica* twigs and flowers are used as a remedy for diarrhea (Perry and Metzger, 1980). *Tamarix ericoides* has been used in folk medicine for the treatment of asthma (Khyade *et al.*, 2010). *Tamarix manna* is used in medicine in India and Arabia (Hutchinson, 1967). The twigs of *Tamarix dioica* are used in local medicines for curing ring worms, gonorrhea (Said, 1969). The leaves of *Tamarix hispida* are used in traditional medicine in the treatment of dysentery, rheumatism, and ulcers (Sokolov, 1986). *Tamarix troupii* is an ornamental plant and is used in medicine and in tanning (Chopra *et al.*, 1956).

### 2.3.2. Folk medicinal uses of the genus *Myricaria*

The branches and leaves of the genus *Myricaria* are used in the folk medicine for treatment of cold, asthema, measles, scorpion poison, and for limiting the effects of poison (Zhao *et al.*, 2005a). *Myricaria Laxiflora* is a rare and endangered riparian shrub in Three Gorges zone, China. Locally, the plants are widely used as a traditional herbal medicine for scald and arthritis.(Wei *et al.*, 2012). *Myricaria longifolia* is used in traditional Mongolian medicine to heal fever, poisoning and liver diseases. It is an ingredient of various prescriptions consisting of several herbal components. (Obmann *et al.*, 2010).

### 2.3.3. Folk medicinal uses of *Myricaria germanica:*

The bark extract of *M. germanica* has been used in folk medicine for jaundice, while the infusion of the leaves was used as analgesic and was found to possess antimicrobial activity and to control chronic bronchitis (Kirbag *et al.*, 2009b; Phani *et al.*, 2009). In addition to, the juice extracted from fresh young shoots with tender leaves is used as one of ingredients in the medicines to cure joint pains.(Singh, 2012).

### 2.3.4. *Myricaria germanica* in Tibetan medicine:

Tibetan medicine is a centuries-old traditional medical system that employs a complex approach to diagnosis, incorporating techniques such as pulse analysis and urinalysis and utilizes behavior and dietary modification, medicines composed of natural materials (e.g., herbs and minerals) and physical therapies (e.g. Tibetan acupuncture, etc.) to treat illness.

*M.germanica* is a maim component of many Tibetan composition for treatment of different illness and many other medicinal purposes (Clark and Lama, 1995).

*M.germanica* can be used for manufacturing whitening antiaging cosmetics (Zhang *et al.*, 2012), Tibetan medicine used for treating central neurogenic pains with advantages of strong analgesic effect. (Baima *et al.*, 2011). A product with Fe content not less than 7.0% can be used for treating iron-deficiency anemia, protecting liver, detoxifying liver. It has the advantages of stable quality, good therapeutic effect (Duo, 2011).

Tibetan medicine comprises *M. germanica*, is used for treating bone fracture, with no use of chemical stabilizers and no toxic adverse effects (Zhang *et al.*, 2011a).

Traditional Chinese medicine composition is manufactured from *M. germanica* and other herbs can be used for treating bronchial asthma, and has the advantages of good curative effect, no stabilizer, and no toxic or side effect (Li *et al.*, 2011), A traditional Chinese medicine composition can be used for treating insufficiency in cerebral blood supply, and has the advantages of good curative effect, no stabilizer (Wang *et al.*, 2011).

Tibetan medicine aerosol is prepared from *M. germanica* as a main component The Tibetan medicine aerosol may be used for treating acute/chronic sprain, contusion, lumbar muscle strain, trauma, pain, hyperosteogeny, stiff neck, periarthritis humeroscapularis, rheumatosis and rheumatoid disease, with advantages of advanced formulation, simple process and quick action (Li and Liu, 2009).

Tibetan medicine is prepared mainly from *Panax ginseng* and *M. germanica*. The composition can be processed into tablet, capsule or granule for treating tinea pedis and tinea manus (He, 2009).

The medical toothpaste is prepared mainly from Gypsum Rubrum, pearl powder and *M. germanica*. The medical toothpaste has antiinflammatory, hemostatic, analgesic and repercussive effects (Lei *et al.*, 2008b). Another medicated toothpaste comprises *Lamiophlomis rotata, Margarita, M. germanica, Oxytropi*s, and matrix 75-88%. The toothpaste can be used for cleaning and caring oral cavity. It has analgesic, hemostatic, anti-inflammatory and antibacterial effects; and has preventive and therapeutic effect on oral diseases such as gingival hemorrhage, gingivitis, periodontitis, gingival atrophy and oral ulcer (Lei *et al.*, 2008a).

The composition of medicated drink contains plants selected from *M. germanica* and other herbs in addition to vitamin B. Ingestion of the drink by 40-65-yrears old female volunteers reduced sleepiness and fatigue and increased motivation (Yamamoto *et al.*, 2007a).

Tibetan cream, toning lotion and emulsion containing *M. germanica* has moisture keeping effect, and can improve and prevent skin roughness (Yamamoto *et al.*, 2007b).

A Chinese medicinal composition for medicated bath, is prepared mainly from *Artemisiae, Ephedrae,* and *M. germanicae*. The composition has effects in relieving exterior syndrome, inducing perspiration, relieving pain and inflammation, reducing yellow water, and promoting blood circulation for removing obstruction in collaterals, and is suitable for various dermatogic disease, rheumarthritis, rheumatoid arthritis, gout, hemiplegia, puerperal diseases and soft tissue sprain (Jiumei, 2006)) The bath salt has effects of protecting health, preventing rheumatism, relieving anxiety, improving sleep, reducing wt., caring skin, enhancing immunity, alleviating inflammation, resisting fatigue, promoting metab., blood circulation, and blood flow, supplementing energy, resisting wind-cold, and eliminating summer heat (Lei and Zhang, 2005)

A patch is prepared from *M.germanica* in addition to other herbs can be used for treating various cancers, such as ovarian cancer, pulmonary carcinoma, hepatocarcinoma, and bladder cancer (Zhang, 2005).

Tibetan medicinal oral or topical dosage forms comprising mainly *Curcuma* Rhizome, and *M. germanica*. The composition has effects in promoting blood circulation, removing blood stasis, relaxing muscles and tendons, expelling collateral obstruction, and relieving swelling and pain. It can be used to treat acute and chronic sprain and contusion, rheumatism, rheumatoid diseases, scapulohumeral periarthritis, osteoarthritis, hyperosteogeny, arthritis, and acute and chronic soft tissue injury (Lei, 2005).

Tibetan medicinal composition (hepatitis B treating capsule) is prepared from: *M.germanicae* and othe herbs) The composition has heat clearing away, dampness removing, depressed liver-dispersing, spleen function regulating, blood stasis relieving, antiinflammatory, and function of gallbladder promoting effects; and can be used for the treatment of acute or chronic hepatitis, alc. Hepatic disease, fatty liver, and hepatitis B (Jiumei, 2001).

Tibetan medicinal composition Bath Lotion, is containing mainly *M. germanicae*, *Artemisiae sieversianae*, *Xanthoceratis*, and Herba *Ephedrae*; The product can be used through steam bath or bath to treat rheumatic arthritis, rheumatoid arthritis, chronic pain of low back and legs, and dermatoses (Ai *et al.*, 2000).

Tibetan powder comprises hot extracting natural Chinese medicinal material (such as *M. germanicae* and other herbs). The powered medicine can be used for treating arthralgia syndrome, rheumatism, rheumatoid diseases and dermatoses. (Lei *et al.*, 1999)

## 2.4. BIOLOGICAL ACTIVITY

### 2.4.1. Biological activities of *Myricaria* species:

Early studies have shown that several oligomeric ellagitannins exhibit in *vivo* antitumor activity against sarcoma 180 and MM2 in mice, which was attributed to an enhanced host immune response (Miyamoto *et al.*, 1987; Miyamoto *et al.*, 1993b). In another study, oligomeric ellagitannins exhibited *in vivo* antitumor (against S-180 in mice) and in vitro cytotoxic (against cancer cell lines) activities; thus, direct cytotoxicity and host-mediated antitumor mechanisms were suggested (Wang *et al.*, 1999). Recently, *in vitro* studies conducted with tumor cell lines have shown that several monomeric, dimeric, and oligomeric ellagitannins and their building units, the gallic and ellagic acids, exhibit potent cytotoxicity against carcinoma cell lines and lower cytotoxicity to normal cells (Ito *et al.*, 2000; Sakagami *et al.*, 2000; Yang *et al.*, 2000; Zunino and Capranico, 1997).

The phytochemical screening of *M. elegans* Royle (Tamaricaceae) led to the isolation of six terpenes from the chloroform fraction. These compounds were suggested by the researchers to be responsible for the mild sedative activity of the plant. (Edewor-Kuponiyi, 2013). The *in vivo* antinociceptive investigation of *M. elegans* showed a significant increase in the tail-flick latency, accompanied by mild sedation and severe ataxia. Considering the known activities of some of the compounds isolated from the plant, it may be hypothesized that the increase in the tail-flick latency may be the combined effect of analgesia, ataxia, and sedation, rather than analgesia alone. These findings suggest *M. elegans* to be a potential source for activity-guided isolation of important natural compounds with a variety of effects (Khan *et al.*, 2010). Two pentacyclic triterpenes eleganene-A (1) and eleganene-B isolated from *M. elegans* exhibited significant antibacterial activity (Ahmad *et al.*, 2008). Eighty percent methanol extract of *M. elegans* Royle showed *in vitro* inhibition of acetylcholinesterase, butyrylcholinesterase and lipoxygenase (Ahmad *et al.*, 2003).

The ethyl acetate fraction obtained from the whole herb extract of *M. alopecuroides* exhibited a particularly potent antibacterial activity especially against *S. aureus* and *M. luteus*, in comparison to the *n*- butanol and dichloromethane fractions (zone of inhibition for both microorganism 16.4 mm). (MIC) of crude ethanol extract of *M. alopecuroides* were 2 mg/disc against the two microorganisms under investigation, respectively. (Enkhmaa *et al.*, 2008). Ethyl acetate fraction of *M. alopecoroides* exhibited also a potential acetylcholinesterase, poly(ADP-ribose) polymerase, malondialdehyde inhibitory effects and *P. aeruginosa*, *E. coli*, *E. faecalis*, *S. aureus* and *M. luteus* antimicrobial activity.(Gendaram *et al.*, 2008).

Aqueous extract of *M. longifolia* have been shown to inhibit the growth of liver carcinoma cells (HepG$_2$), breast cancer cells (MCF-7), and primary rat hepatocytes. The same extract caused damage of the isolated rat liver during perfusion experiments.(Obmann *et al.*, 2010).

Gallicin, gallic acid derivative, isolated from *M. Laxiflora* showed obvious antimicrobial activities. The minimum inhibitory concentration MIC of this compound was 5 mg/ml against *S. aureus* and *Rhizopus*, and 10 mg/ml against *E. coli*. Furthermore, just like propyl gallate, gallicin showed fairly active for oxidation resistance in the presence of $H_2O_2$.(Wei *et al.*, 2012).

Two new pentacyclic triterpenoids myricarin A and B (1 and 2) isolated from the stems of *M. paniculata*, showed promising cytotoxic activities against several different cell lines (Li *et al.*, 2005).

## 2.4.2. Biological activities of *Myricaria germanica*:

The Methanol extract of *M. germanica* showed promising antimicrobial activity against *P.aeruginosa*, *S.aureus* , *C.albicans* , *B.subtilis S.epidermis* . The antibacterial spectrum of *M.germanica* seems closer to reference antibiotic Kanamycin. In addition, the methanol extract of *M. germanica* imparted significant cellular cytotoxic effects using Sulpharhodamine-B assay on different human cancer cell lines namely THP-1 (Leukemia), A-549 (Lung), HCT-15 (Colon), Cervix (Hela) and Prostrate (PC-3) . However, the most promising results were obtained against Leukemia (THP-1), Colon (HCT-15) and Lung (A549) cancer cell lines. (Mubashir, 2011; Mubashir *et al.*, 2010 ).

*In vitro* antimicrobial activities of extracts of six plant and standard antibiotic Streptomysin sulfate and Nystatin were evaluated. The extract of *M. germanica* did not show any activity against *P. aeruginosa, E. coli, P.vulgaris, S. aureus, C. albicans* while antimicrobial activity was observed against *B.megaterium, K. pneumoniae, C. glabrata, C. tropicalis* (inhibition zone between 8- 18 mm), relative to the standards (9-11mm). (Kirbag *et al.*, 2009a).

# 3. MATERIALS, APPARATUS AND METHODS

## 3.1. Materials:

### 3.1.1. Plant materials:

Fresh aerial parts of *Myricaria germanica* (L) Desv (Tamaricaceae) were collected in June (2009) from the botanical garden of the University Bonn, Germany and identified by Dr. Peter König, Botanical garden, Ernst-Moritz-Arndt-University Greifswald, Germany. A Voucher specimen is deposited at the herbarium of the N.R.C. (CAIRO).

## 3.2. Phytochemical screening:

### General tests for preliminary screening of phyto-constituents

### 3.2.1. Flavonoids:

**Shinoda' s test** (Geissman, 1966)

Few drops of hydrochloric acid were added to an ethanolic extract, followed by few mg of magnesium turnings. A red or pink color indicated the presence of flavonoids.

### 3.2.2. Coumarines (Farnsworth, 1954)

A small amount of moistened plant sample was placed in a test tube. The tube was covered with a filter paper moistened with a dilute solution of sodium hydroxide. The covered test tube was then placed in a boiling water bath for several minutes; the paper is removed and exposed to UV light. A yellow green fluorescence indicated the presence of coumarins.

### 3.2.3. Steroids and/ or triterpenoids:

**Liebermann- Burchard's test** (Leiber mann and Burchard, 1890)

To a chlorophormic solution of the extract, 0.3 ml of acetic anhydride and few drops of concentrated sulphuric acid were added along the side of the tube. A reddish violet color at the junction of the two layers indicated the presence of sterols.

### 3.2.4. Carbohydrates and / or glycosides:

**Molisch' test** (Molisch, 1886)

Two ml of the aqueous extract were mixed with 0.2 ml of the ethanolic α- naphthol (20%) and 2 ml sulphuric acid along the side of the test tube to form 2 layers. A violet zone at the junction of the 2 layers indicated the presence of carbohydrates.

### 3.2.5. Saponins (Gonzales and Delango, 1962)
**Froth test**

One gm of the plant sample was boiled in 10 ml water for a few minutes, filtered and shaked. A persistent froth indicated the presence of saponins.

### 3.2.6. Phenolics (Trease, 1966)
**Ferric chloride test**

Nine gm of ferric chloride were dissolved in water and completed to 100 ml. 1 ml of this reagent was added to the aqueous acidified extract. Condensed tannins gave a green color while hydrolysable tannins gave a blue –black color.

### 3.2.7. Alkaloids (Fulton, 1932)
**Mayers' reagent**

One gm of mercuric chloride in 60 ml water was added to a solution of 5 gm of potassium iodide in 20 ml water. Completed to 100 ml solution with sufficient water. 3 drops of this reagent were added to the residue of an alcoholic extract dissolved in 1 ml dil. Hcl. The formation of turbidity or precipitate indicated the presence of alkaloids.

### 3.2.8. Anthraquinones (Fairbrain, 1942)
**2.8.1. Borntraeger's test (for anthraquinone aglycone)**

The powdered material was macerated in an immiscible organic solvent. After filteration, aqueous ammonia or caustic soda was added and shaked. A red coloration in the aqueous layer indicated the presence of anthraquinone aglycone.

**2.8.2. Modified Borntraeger' s test (for anthraquinone glycosides)**

The powdered material was first hydrolyzed with alcoholic potassium hydroxide and further treated as in Borntraeger's test. A rose red color in the aqueous layer indicated the presence of anthraquinone glycosides.

## 3.3. Phytochemical investigation of *Myricaria germanica* (L) Desv (Tamaricaceae)

### 3.3.1. Plant extract:

The fresh *M. germanica* leaves (800 g) were homogenized in EtOH–H$_2$O (3:1) mixture (three extractions each with 1 L). The solvent was removed under reduced pressure at $\approx 45°$ C. The process yielded finally 150 g of a sticky dark brown material.

### 3.3.2. Authentic reference materials

Authentic samples of the known flavonols quercetin, kaempferol, tamarixitin together with authentic samples of phenolic carboxylic acids, e.g. gallic or ellagic acids, also, commonly occurring sugars and phenolics were used for comparative paper chromatography. The samples are provided from the laboratory of phytochemistry and plant systematic, NRC.

### 3.3.3. Chromatographic materials

#### 3.3.3.1. Paper chromatography

Sheets of Whatman paper No 1 or 3 MM were used for two dimensional, comparative or preparative paper chromatography.

#### 3.3.3.2. Solvent systems for paper chromatography

The chromatographic solvents used are abbreviated by the symbols given (Table 2).

**Table (2): Solvent systems for paper chromatography**

| Symbol | Composition | Percent by v |
|---|---|---|
| 1- BAW | *n*- butanol / acetic acid / water | 4 : 1 : 5 (upper phase) |
| 2- H$_2$O | water | |
| 3- 6 % ACOH | acetic acid / water | 0.6 : 9.4 |
| 4- 15 % ACOH | acetic acid / water | 1.5: 8.5 |
| 5- BBPW | benzene / *n*-butanol / pyridine / water | 1 : 5 : 3 : 3 (upper phase) |

### 3.3.3.3. Column chromatography

The separation of phenolic and flavonoids components was performed by column fractionation of the extract or its fractions on one of the following stationary phases as stated in each case.

a. Polyamide powder, polyamide 6-S for column chromatography. Riedel-De Haen AG, Seelze- Hannover, Germany.

b. Sephadex LH-20 (25-100 µm), Pharmacia fine chemicals.

### 3.3.3.4. Solvent system for column chromatography

a. Gradient concentration of $MeOH/H_2O$.

b. *n*-Butanol water saturated.

c. Methanol: Benzene: Bidistilled $H_2O$ in the ratio 60:38:2.

### 3.3.3.5. Spray reagents and test solutions

**Specific for phenolic compounds**

a. Ferric chloride (1 % methanolic solution) (Neich, 1960)

b. Gibb's reagent (Neich, 1960)

 i- A freshly prepared N-2, 6-trichlorobenzoquinone-4-monoimine, (0.5% methanol solution

 ii- Saturated aqueous sodium bicarbonate solution.

**Specific for galloyl esters**

Potassium iodate $KIO_3$ (saturated aqueous solution) (Haddock *et al.*, 1982)

**Specific for hexahydroxydiphenoyl esters**

Nitrous acid (Gupta *et al.*, 1982): To a volume of 100 ml ice cold aqueous $NaNO_2$ solution (10 %) few drops (5-10) of glacial acetic acid are added, the spray is used immediately after preparation.

**Specific for flavonoids**

a. Aluminium chloride (Wender and Gage, 1949) (1 % methanolic solution). Chromatograms sprayed with $AlCl_3$ were air dried then observed in visible and under UV light to note any change in color.

b. Diphenyl borinic acid ethanol amine ester (Pachaly *et al.*, 1990), (Naturstoff reagent).

 i - 1% Diphenylboryloxyethyl amine in MeOH .

ii - 5% polyethyleneglycol 400 in ethanol.

Inspection of the dry chromatograms after 30 minutes under UV light at 365 nm.

**Specific for carboxylic acids**

Aniline / xylose ((Harborne, 1973; Smith, 1976), the chromatograms have to be heated at 105°C for 4-5 minutes.

**Specific for sugars**

a. Aniline / hydrogen phthalate (Jurd, 1962), the chromatograms have to be heated at 105°C for 4-5 min.

b. *p*-Anisidine phosphate (Mukkerjee and Srivasttava, 1952), the chromatograms have to be heated at 105°C for 4-5 min.

**Reagents for UV spectrophotometric analysis of flavonoids** (Harborne and William, 1975; Mabry *et al.*, 1969)

1- Sodium methoxide: Freshly cut of metallic sodium (2.5g) is added cautiously in small pieces to 100 ml of dry methanol.

2- Aluminium chloride: Anhydrous aluminium chloride (5g) is cautiously added to 100 ml of methanol.

3- Hydrochloric acid: Hydrochloric acid (5ml) is mixed with 15 ml distilled water.

4- Sodium acetate: Anhydrous coarsely powdered sodium acetate.

5- Boric acid: Anhydrous powdered boric acid.

### 3.4. Materials for biological study

### 3.4.1. Chemicals and drugs:

Sulfarhodamine, trypsin-EDTA, phosphate buffered saline (PBS), trichloroacetic acid (TCA), glacial acetic acid and tris-HCl were purchased from Sigma Chemical Co. (St. Louis, MO). RPMI-164 media, fetal bovine serum and other cell culture materials were purchased from ATCC (Houston, TX, USA). Other reagents were of the highest analytical grade.

**Concentration scheme of SRB assay reagents**

| Reagent | Concentration |
|---|---|
| Sulforhodamine B Solution | 0.4% in 1% Acetic Acid |
| Trichloroacetic Acid (Fixative Solution) | 50% |
| Acetic Acid Solution (Wash Solution) | 10% |
| Tris Base Solution (Solubilization Solution) | 10 mM |

### 3.4.2. Human tumor cell lines for cytotoxic activity:

- *MCF7* ( Breast adenocarcinoma cell line).
- *Huh-7* (Human hepatocellular carcinoma cell line).
- PC-3 (Prostate adenocarcinoma cell line).

Cell lines were obtained from the Egyptian National Cancer Institute, Cairo, Egypt and Max Plank Institute, Heidelberg, Germany. Cells were maintained in RPMI-1640 supplemented with 100 µg/ml streptomycin, 100 units/ml penicillin and 10% heat-inactivated fetal bovine serum in a humidified, 5% (v/v) $CO_2$ atmosphere at 37 °C.

### 3.5. APPARATUS:

3.5.1. Rotary evaporator (Buchi, G, Swizerland).

3.5.2. Ultra-Violet lamp for location of fluorescent spots on chromatograms and bands on columns (6 watt S/W and L/W, VL, France).

3.5.3. Ultra-Violet spectrophotometer (UV recording were made on a Shimadzu UV-Visible-1601 spectrophotometer).

3.5.4. Open glass columns.

3.5.5. Rectangular glass jars of different size and micro-pipette for spotting.

3.5.6. Nuclear Magnetic Resonance Spectrometer, Joel ECA-500 MHz NMR spectrometer, Tokyo, Japan.

3.5.7. Inverted microscope, Olympus 1x70, Tokyo, Japan.

3.5.8. Orbital shaker, OS 20. Boeco, Germany, at 1600 rpm.

3.5.9. Spectrophotometer ELIZA microplate reader, ChroMate-4300, FL, USA.

3.5.10 High resolution ESI mass spectra were measured using a Finnigan LTQ, FT Ultra mass spectrometer (Thermo Fisher Scientific, Bremen, Germany)

## 3.6. Phytochemical methods:
### 3.6.1. Chromatographic methods
#### 3.6.1.1. Paper chromatographic analysis

Paper chromatography was carried out on unwashed Whatman paper No.1 sheets, spotted with the material under investigation and then developed by the respective solvent systems (Table 2). The developed chromatograms were air dried, examined in V and under long and short UV light, then exposed for 2-3 minutes to ammonia vapour (except in case of sugars) and were immediately observed to note the possible changes that may eventually appear in color or fluorescence in visible or UV light. For preparative paper chromatography, Whatman paper No. 3 MM was used. After development of the Whatman paper No.1 chromatograms, the separated flavonoids, phenolics or sugars were detected on the dried chromatograms by spraying with chromogenic spray reagents specific for flavonoids, phenolics or sugar materials.

#### 3.6.1.2. Column chromatographic analysis
**i- Adsorbents**

The isolation and purification of compounds were achieved through the application of the investigated extract or its fractions on one of the stationary phases discussed in section **B-5.**, as stated in each case.

## ii. Technique

After packing the column thoroughly with the stationary phases, a relatively concentrated clear solution of the material under investigation was applied to the top of the column. Elution was then started with selected solvents. The bands developed during the chromatographic process were located under both V and UV lights to note their color and migration with the solvents. Each fraction desorbed from the column as controlled under UV light was then collected and dried under reduced pressure. The fraction or sub-fraction thus received was paper chromatographically analyzed and separately investigated.

### 3.6.1.3. Thin Layer Chromatography:

TLC was carried out for isolated compounds (silica gel) alongside with authentic samples to check out the purity of the isolated compounds using the solvent systems mentioned previously (Table 2).

### 3.6.1.4. Electrophoretic analysis:

Paper electrophoresis was carried out on unwashed Whatman paper No. 3 MM sheet and spotted with the material. The separation of the ionic constituents was effected by an electric field (250 V, 10 mA) and the migration took place in 2.5% Formic acid plus 8% Acetic acid for 90 minutes. After the separation the paper was completely dried and the phenolics were detected with ferric chloride (1% alcoholic solution).

### 3.6.2. Chemical methods

### 3.6.2.1. Complete (Normal) acid hydrolysis

Complete or normal acid hydrolysis was carried out for 2 hours at $100°C$ using aqueous 2 N hydrochloric acid. These conditions could be changed according to the chemical nature of the investigated compound as stated in each case. The hydrolysate was then extracted with ethyl acetate and the received extract was subjected to paper chromatographic investigation alongside with authentic samples. The aqueous layer was then carefully extracted with N-methyl dioctylamine (10% in $CHCl_3$). The acid-free aqueous layer was concentrated under vacuum then co-chromatographed alongside with authentic sugars using solvent system 5 (BBPW). Aniline phthalate spray reagent was then used to detect sugar spots (Vogel, 2001).

### 3.6.2.2. Mild (Controlled) acid hydrolysis

Mild or controlled acid hydrolysis in 0.1 N aqueous hydrochloric acid at 100° C was carried out for 30 minutes. These conditions could be changed according to the chemical nature of the investigated compound as stated in each case. The reaction mixture was examined every 3 minutes by paper chromatographic analysis to detect any intermediates that might be formed. The solvent systems used were 1(BAW), 2 ($H_2O$) and 3(ACOH-6) (Vogel, 2001).

### 3.6.2.3. Enzymatic hydrolysis

Enzymic hydrolysis were done with $\beta$-glucosidase, $\beta$-galactosidase, $\beta$-glucurunosidase or $\alpha$-rhamnosidase at pH 5.2 and 37°C in dark, for 24 hours, the hydrolysate was then extracted with ethyl acetate and the extract received was subjected to paper chromatographic investigation alongside with authentic samples.

### 3.7. Physical methods

#### 3.7.1. UV analysis:

UV recording were made on a Shimadzu UV-Visible-1601 spectrophotometer.

#### 3.7.2. $^1H$ and $^{13}C$- NMR analysis:

Jeol ECA 500 MHz NMR Spectrometer, (National research center, Cairo). $^1H$ chemical shifts ($\delta$) were measured in ppm, relative to TMS and $^{13}C$-NMR chemical shifts to $CD_3(2)CO$ and converted to TMS scale by adding 30 or to DMSO-$d_6$ and converted to TMS scale by adding 39.5 as stated in each case. Typical conditions: spectral width = 8 KHz for $^1H$ and 30 KHz for $^{13}C$, 64 K data points and a flip angle of 45°.

#### 3.7.3. Mass spectrometric analysis:

High resolution ESI mass spectra were measured using a Finnigan LTQ FT Ultra mass spectrometer (Thermo Fisher Scientific, Bremen, Germany) equipped with a Nanomate ESI interface (Advion). An electrospray voltage of 1.7 kV (+ /-) and a transfer capillary temperature of 200 °C were applied. Collision induced dissociation (CID) was performed in the iontrap using a normalized collision energy of 35%, activation time 30 ms, 0.25 activation Q and a precursor ion isolation width of 2 amu. High resolution product ions were detected in the Fourier transform ion cyclotron resonance (FTICR) cell of the mass spectrometer.

Other mass spectra were measured on a Mass spectrometer MAT 95 (Finnigan MAT, Bremen, Germany).

### 3.7.4. Flame atomic absorption analysis:

Flame atomic absorption analysis was performed on a Varian Spectra-AA220 instrument, lamp current: 5 ma, fuel: acetylene, oxidant: air, slitwidth: 0.5 nm.

### 3.7.5. $[\alpha]_D^{27}$ recording:

Optical rotations were obtained by a Kruess P 8000 digital polarimeter.

## 3.8. Methods for the Biological Investigation of the Aqueous Ethanol Extract of *Myricaria germanica*, its column chromatographic fractions and isolated compounds

### Study design

Cell lines: three different solid tumor cell lines were used; breast cancer (MCF-7), prostate (PC-3), and liver (Huh-7) cancer cell.

The following parameters were measured in all tested cell lines:

1. Viability concentration-response curve of the crude extract, fractions and isolated compounds were determined for 72 h using SRB viability assay.
2. Effect of isolated compounds on the cell cycle distribution using DNA cytometric analysis.
3. Activity of caspase-3 as a tool of assessing apoptosis.
4. PARP enzyme activity as a tool of assessing cytotoxic sensitizing ability of the crude extract and its promising isolated fraction.

### 3.8.1. Cell culture

Cells were maintained in RPMI-1640 supplemented with 100 μg/mL streptomycin, 100 units/mL penicillin and 10% heat-inactivated fetal bovine serum in a humidified, 5% (v/v) $CO_2$ atmosphere at 37 °C (Moore *et al.*, 1958).

**Chemicals and reagents:**

**A) RPMI 1640 medium**

| | |
|---|---|
| RPMI 1640 powder | 1 pack for 1X |
| $NaHCO_3$ | 2 g |
| Pyruvate sodium salt | 0.11g |
| 20 mM HEPES | 4.77g |
| Penicillin G | 0.06g |
| Streptomycin sulfate | 0.1g |
| NaOH 1 N | Q.S. to pH=7.4 |
| Autoclaved DDW, ad., 1.0L | |

Sterilize by filtration and store at 4°C

**B) Phosphate Buffered Saline (PBS)**

| | |
|---|---|
| NaCl | 8.00g |
| KCl | 0.20g |
| Na2HPO4. (2H2O) | 1.15g (1.44g) |
| KH2PO4. (12H2O) | 0.20g (2.895g) |
| CaCl2 | 0.1g |
| MgCl2.6H2O | 0.1g |
| HCl | Q.S. to pH 7.4 |
| Autoclaved DDW, ad., 1.0L | |

Sterilize by autoclaving and store at 4°C

**Standard operating procedures:**

**Cell line stock reconstitution:**

1. Cell line stock vial (directly withdrawn from the Liquid $N_2$) was rapidly thawed with a minimal amount of medium (around 1 ml).
2. Reconstituted vial was diluted with 10 ml medium and centrifuged at 1000 rpm for 5 min at 4°C.

3. The supernatant was discarded and the pellet was reconstituted in 1 ml medium, plated in one 150 Ø Petri dish or T-75 flask using 10- 20 ml medium.
4. After 2 days of growth (before 90% confluent), cells were subcultured again in T-75 flask

**Routine subculture procedures**
1. Cells were incubated at 37°C till less than 90% confluent (contact inhibition and change in the morphology takes place in over confluent cultures)
2. The medium were aspirated and cells were washed with PBS pH 7.4.
3. Two ml trypsin/EDTA (0.25%) were added into the culture plate until cell detachment (Inverted microscope guided) and then tapped gently.
4. The cells were harvested with 10% FBS containing media (10 ml in case of 75-T flask) and centrifuged at 1000 rpm for 5 min at 4°C
5. The supernatant was discarded and the pellet was reconstituted in 3 ml medium.
6. Reconstituted cells were directly distributed into 3 new plates 150 Ø Petri dish or T-75 flask using 10- 20 ml medium.

## 3.8.2. Sulforhodamine B colorimetric assay for evaluation of cytotoxicity (Vichai and Kirtikara, 2006)

**Assay principle**

The assay relies on the ability of SRB to bind to protein components of cells that have been fixed to culture plates by trichloroacetic acid (TCA). SRB is a bright-pink aminoxanthene dye with two sulfonic groups that bind to basic amino-acid residues under mild acidic conditions, and dissociate under basic conditions. As the binding of SRB is stoichiometric, the amount of dye extracted from stained cells is directly proportional to the cell mass.

The cytotoxicity of crude extract and isolated fractions was tested against MCF-7, PC-3 and Huh-7 cells by SRB assay. Exponentially growing cells were collected using 0.25% Trypsin-EDTA and plated in 96-well plates at 1000-2000 cells/well. Cells were exposed to the extract or isolated fractions for 72 h and subsequently fixed with TCA (10%) for 1 h at 4 °C. After several washings, cells were exposed to 0.4% SRB solution for 10 min in dark place and subsequently washed with 1% glacial acetic acid. After overnight drying, Tris-HCl was used to dissolve the SRB-stained cells and color intensity was measured at 540 nm with microplate reader (Skehan *et al.*, 1990).

**Chemicals and reagents:**
RPMI1640 media
Trypsin-EDTA (0.25%)
PBS
TCA
SRB (0.4%)
Glacial acetic acid (1%)
10 mM Tris-HCl

**Procedures**

**Cell seeding for SRB Assay (original monolayer 96-well plate seeding):**
1. Cells under investigation were trypsinized and proper dilution in the compatible medium was made.
2. Aliquots of 100 µl cell suspension containing 1000 cell were seeded into flat bottom 96-well plate (according to the cell line doubling time, and operator handling usually range from 500-2000 cell per well).
3. Plates were incubated in a humidified 37 °C, 5% $CO_2$ chamber for 24 hr.
4. Another aliquots of 100µl media containing the drug conc. range (1 ng/ml to 100 µg/ml) under investigation were added to treated lanes, and blank media to the +ve, and –ve control lanes. (N.B.#3: this is considered the zero time for treatment)
5. Plates were incubated in a humidified 37 °C, 5% $CO_2$ chamber for another 72 hrs. (N.B. 4: for the long incubation period the media might need to be changed, and some time PBS washing is recommended according to the treatment under investigation).

**SRB assay procedure: (for simple 96 well plate format)**
1. On the day of analysis, the 96 well plates were centrifuged at 1000 rpm, 4 °C, and for 5 min.
2. The media containing the drug solution were removed.
3. **Fixation:** 150 µl of 10% TCA were added, and the plates were incubated at 4 °C for 1 h.
4. The fixative solution was removed and washed 5 times with DDW
5. Aliquots of 70 µl of 0.4 % SRB solution were added and incubated for 10 min at RT in a dark place

6. Plates were washed 3 times with 1% acetic acid, and let to air-dry over night
7. To dissolve SRB-bound protein, aliquots of 150 µl of 10 mM Tris-HCl were added and shaken for 2 min
8. Immediately measure the absorbance at 540 nm

**Data analysis**

The viability dose response curve of compounds was analyzed using $E_{max}$ model (Eq. 1).

$$\% \text{ Cell viability} = (100 - R) \times \left(1 - \frac{[D]^m}{K_d^m + [D]^m}\right) + R \quad \ldots\ldots\ldots\ldots \text{(Eq. 1)}$$

Where R is the residual unaffected fraction (the resistance fraction), [D] is the drug concentration used, $K_d$ is the drug concentration that produces a 50% reduction of the maximum inhibition rate and m is a Hill-type coefficient. $IC_{50}$ was defined as the drug concentration required to reduce optical density to 50% of that of the control (i.e., $K_d = IC_{50}$ when R=0 and $E_{max}$ =100-R) (Skehan et al., 1990).about abrev.

### 3.8.3. Determination of caspase-3 activity

**Assay principle**

Human Active Caspase-3 Quantikine ELISA Kit uses a biotinylated caspase inhibitor to covalently modify the large subunit of caspase-3. Inhibitor is added directly to the culture medium where it enters apoptotic cells and forms a stable thio-ether bond with the cysteine on the active site of the enzyme. Inhibitor does not covalently modify inactive caspase-3, which is the basis for discrimination between active and inactive caspase-3. Cells are then solubilized in a denaturing extraction buffer and diluted to reduce denaturant concentration. Specific detection of active caspase-3 utilizes a quantitative sandwich enzyme immunoassay technique. A monoclonal antibody specific for caspase-3 has been pre-coated onto a 96-well plate. Cell extract samples containing covalently linked active caspase-3-biotin-ZVKD are pipetted into the wells and any caspase-3 present (active or inactive) is captured by the immobilized antibody. Inactive caspase-3 zymogen is not modified by the biotin-ZVKD-FMK inhibitor and therefore is not detected. Following a wash to remove any unbound substances, streptavidin conjugated to horseradish peroxidase is added to the wells and binds to the biotin on the inhibitor. Following a wash to remove any unbound Streptavidin-HRP reagent, a substrate solution is added to the wells. The enzyme reaction yields a blue product that turns yellow when the Stop Solution is added. The intensity of the color measured is in proportion to the amount of active caspase-3 bound in the initial step. The ELISA measures the relative amount of caspase-3 large subunit modified with biotin-ZVKD-FMK. Since the modification requires that the large subunit is present in an active caspase-3, the amount of active caspase-3 is directly proportional to the amount of biotin-ZVKD-FMKmodified large subunit. The sample values are then read off the standard curve.

**Chemical and reagents**

Active Caspase-3 Microplate
Active Caspase-3 Conjugate Concentrate
Type 12 Conjugate Diluent
Active Caspase-3 Standard
Calibrator Diluent RD5-20 Concentrate (5X)
Extraction Buffer Concentrate (5X)
Biotin-ZVKD-fmk Inhibitor
Wash Buffer Concentrate
Color Reagent A
Color Reagent B
Stop Solution

**Procedures**

**A) Labeling of active caspases in cells**

After treatment, 2 µl of 5 mM biotin-ZVKD-fmk were added per 1 mL of culture medium to obtain a final concentration of 10 µM. Cells were incubated with the biotin-ZVKD-fmk inhibitor for 1 h.

## Preparation of cell extracts

1. Media containing detached cells were removed and saved.
2. Cells were gently washed with PBS; collected and pooled with the wash.
3. Attached cells were scraped into Extraction Buffer (1X) containing protease inhibitors using 1 mL per $1 \times 10^7$ cells.
4. Scrapped cells were combined with previous PBS, wash and media and centrifuged at 1000x g for 5 minutes to pellet detached cells. Supernatant was discarded.
5. Pelleted detached cells were suspended in PBS and centrifuge at $1000 \times g$ for 5 minutes Supernatant was discarded.
6. Extract from step 3 was added to the pellet from step 5 and vortexed for 1 minute; allowed to sit for 2 hours at room temperature or overnight at 2-8°C. The extended time in Extraction Buffer (1X) containing protease inhibitors ensures that maximum denaturation is achieved. Samples can be stored in Extraction Buffer for up to 14 days at 2-8°C.
7. Immediately prior to assay, samples were diluted 10-20 fold with Calibrator Diluent RD5-20 (1X). Diluted samples can be stored for 14 days at -20° C.

## B) Dilution of cell extracts

Cell extracts containing $1 \times 10^7$ cells/ml require a final 20-fold dilution in Calibrator Diluent RD5-20 (1X) to obtain $5 \times 10^5$ cells/ml.

## Assay procedure

1. All reagents, standard dilutions, and samples were prepared as directed in the previous sections.
2. Excess microplate strips were removed from the plate frame, returned to the foil pouch containing the desiccant pack, resealed.
3. Standard or samples (100 µl) were added to wells, covered with the adhesive strip provided, incubated for 2 hours at room temperature.
4. Each well was aspirated and washed, repeating the process four times for a total of five washes. Washing was by filling each well with Wash Buffer (400 µL) using a squirt bottle, multi-channel pipette, manifold dispenser or autowasher. Complete removal of liquid at each step is essential for good performance. After the last wash, any remaining Wash Buffer was removed by aspirating or decanting. The plate was inverted and tapped against clean paper towels.

5. Active Caspase-3 Conjugate (100 µL) was added to each well, covered with a new adhesive strip, incubated for 1 hour at room temperature.
6. The aspiration/wash in step 4 was repeated.
7. Substrate Solution (100 µL) was added to each well, incubated for 30 minutes at room temperature **(Protect from light)**.
8. Stop Solution (100 µL) was added to each well, Plate was gently tapped to ensure thorough mixing.
9. Optical density of each well was determined within 30 minutes, using a microplate reader set to 450 nm, readings at 540 nm or 570 nm were subtracted from the readings at 450 nm. This subtraction will correct for optical imperfections in the plate. Readings made directly at 450 nm without correction may be higher and less accurate.

### 3.8.4. Analysis of cell cycle distribution
**Assay principle (BD FACSVerse System User's Guide)**

Measuring DNA content of cells is a well established method for monitoring cell proliferation, cell cycle, and DNA ploidy. Proliferating cells progress through various phases of the cell cycle (G0, G1, S, G2, and M phase). At different stages of the cell cycle, cell nuclei contain different amounts of DNA. After receiving signals for proliferation, diploid cells exit the resting state Gap 0 (G0) phase and enter the Gap 1 (G1) phase. At this stage, the diploid cells maintain their ploidy by retaining two complete sets of chromosomes (2N). As the cells enter the synthesis (S) phase, DNA replication starts, and in this phase, cells contain varying amounts of DNA. The DNA replication continues until the DNA content reaches a tetraploid state (4N) with twice the DNA content of the diploid state. Tetraploid cells in the G2 phase start preparing for division and enter the mitosis (M) phase when the cells divide into two identical diploid (2N) daughter cells. The daughter cells continue on to another division cycle or enter the resting stage (G0 phase). Based on DNA content alone, the M phase is indistinguishable from the G2 phase, and G0 is indistinguishable from G1. Therefore, when based on DNA content, cell cycle is commonly described by the G0/G1, S, and G2/M phases.

The BD Cycletest Plus reagent kit provides a set of reagents to isolate and stain cell nuclei from fresh or previously frozen cell suspensions. Briefly, the procedure involves lysing the cell membrane with a nonionic detergent, eliminating the cell cytoskeleton and nuclear proteins with trypsin, digesting the cellular RNA with Ribonuclease A, and stabilizing the nuclear chromatin with spermine. Propidium iodide (PI) is used to stain the DNA of isolated nuclei in a stoichiometric fashion. PI bound to DNA can be excited by a 488-nm laser and detected using suitable detector. The emitted fluorescence intensity can be measured using a flow cytometer such as the BD FACSVerse system (Becton Dickinson Immunocytometry Systems, San Jose, CA). For each sample, 10,000 events are acquired. Cell cycle distribution is calculated using CELLQuest software (Becton Dickinson Immunocytometry Systems, San Jose, CA).

**Procedure**
1. **Cell harvesting:** perform normal regular trypsinization, but do not discard the collected media keep it to re-neutralize the trypsin, also the media might contain some molecules important for the flow cytometric analysis. Also the PBS used should be ice cold.
2. **Centrifuge (1000-1500 rpm, 5-7 min, 4°C) and remove the supernatant:** do not remove the supernatant completely keep some (about 0.5 ml) to re-suspend the pellets
3. **Cell washing with ice cold PBS:** after pellets resuspension add 10 ml ice cold PBS for cell washing
4. **Centrifuge (1000-1500 rpm, 5-7 min, 4°C) and remove the supernatant:**
5. **Gently re-suspend the pellet in approximately 1ml of ice cold PBS then add another 2 ml**
6. **Fixation:** slowly add 5 ml 70% EthOH/PBS while vortexing. The vortexing is to prevent cell aggregation. The EthOH is used for fixation of DNA. If we are going to perform flow cytometry to study apoptosis; we should fix with paraformaldhyde because paraformaldhyde prevent small DNA molecules from leakage outside the cell.
7. **Keep in ice for 1 h**
8. **Cells may be stored in the fixative solution up to 2 weeks in -20°C**
9. **On the day of analysis:** if the sample is stored you have to melt it in 4°C; then leave in RT for 15 min; followed by vortexing to prevent cell aggregation
10. **Centrifuge (1000-1500 rpm, 5-7 min, 4°C) and remove the supernatant:** do not remove the supernatant completely keep some (about 1 ml) to allow for gradual alc. Conc. Change

11. **Cell washing twice with RT PBS:** do not drain all the supernatant keep one ml for gradual alcohol dilution otherwise cell aggregation will take place due to sudden solvent change.

   Gently re-suspend the pellet in approximately 1 ml staining mix by pipetting
   Staining Mix: A) Add 0.5 ml of RNase (50 µg/ml) + Eth Br 0.625 mg + 24.5 ml PBS to give a final conc. of Eth Br = 25 µg/ml.

   B) Add 0.5 ml of RNase (50 µg/ml) + PI 1.25 mg + 24.5 ml PBS to give a final conc. of PI = 50 µg/ml.
   Add in water bath at 37 °C for 5-20 min; protect from light; and measure on the apparatus.

12. Filter 1 ml PBS through **spectra/mesh Nylon,** N macro-porous filter-woven mesh porosity 5-1000 µm (spectrum laboratory product-CA-USA-tel: 310-885-4600, fax: 310-885-4666), followed by 1 ml sample, immediate prior to measure on the apparatus.

### 3.8.5. Determination of Poly (ADP-ribose) polymerase (PARP) enzyme activity
**Principle**

Poly (ADP-ribosylation) of nuclear proteins is a post-translational event that occurs in response to DNA damage. Poly (ADP-ribose) Polymerase (PARP) is the enzyme catalyzing the NAD-dependent addition of ribose to adjacent nuclear proteins. PARP is an abundant nuclear protein present in all somatic cells. PARP plays an important role in DNA repair. During apoptosis, PARP is specifically cleaved by members of the proteases (e.g. Caspase-3). It is converted to fragments with minimal activity that was not activated by damaged DNA. It appears that PARP cleavage is a mechanism that prevents apoptotic cells from repairing their DNA (Satoh and Lindahl, 1992). The PARP Universal Colorimetric Assay Kit measures the incorporation of biotinylated Poly (ADP-ribose) onto histone proteins in a 96-well plate.

To assess the activity of different isolated fractions to block DNA repair, PARP enzyme activity was assessed using cell free system enzyme assay. Briefly, the remaining PARP enzyme activity was determined after incubation with the pre-determined $IC_{50}$ using PARP Universal Colorimetric Assay (R&D Systems, Minneapolis, USA) according to the manufacturer's instructions. Standard PARP enzyme inhibitor (3-Amino-benzamide) was used against purified PARP enzyme to plot standard curve and the intensity of the color measured in samples are then read off the standard curve.

**Statistical analysis**

Data are presented as mean ± SD. Analysis of variance (ANOVA) with LSD post hoc test was used for testing the significance using SPSS® for windows, version 17.0.0 (SPSS Inc., Chicago, IL, USA). A value of $p<0.05$ was taken as a cut off value for significance.

# 4. PHENOLIC CONSTITUENTS OF THE AERIAL PARTS OF AQUEOUS ALCOHOL EXTRACT OF *Myricaria germanica* (L.) Desv.

## 4.1. Phytochemical screening of the aerial parts of *Myricaria germanica*

The powdered dried sample of the aerial parts of *Myricaria germanica*, was screened for the following constituents: flavonoids, coumarins, sterols and/ or triterpenes, carbohydrates and / or glycosides, saponins, phenolics, alkaloids and anthraquinones following methods for phyto constituents described on pages 26-27.

Results are listed in table (3).

**Table (3): Phytochemical screening of the aerial parts of *Myricaria germanica***

| Constituents | Results |
|---|---|
| Flavonoid , free | +++ |
| combined | + |
| Coumarins | - |
| Sterols and/ or terpenes | + |
| Carbohydratesand / or glycosides | + |
| Saponins | - |
| Phenolics | +++ |
| Alkaloids | - |
| Anthraquinones | - |

From the above given results, it is concluded that the phytochemical constituents of this species contain mainly flavonoids and phenolics.

## 4.2. Extraction:

The method described on page 28, was applied for the preparation of the extract.

### 4.2.1. Qualitative phenolic analysis of the extract:

The following procedures were performed. They include color and precipitation reactions necessary for characterizing plant phenolics. The received results are given in (Table 4).

**Table (4): Qualitative phenolic analysis of extract:**

| Test | The observation | Conclusion |
|---|---|---|
| 1. Gelatin (1% aqueous solution) | white precipitate | Presence of tannins |
| 2. $FeCl_3$ (1% ethanolic solution) | Intense blue color | Presence of phenolics |
| 3. $Pb(CH_3COO)_2$ (10% aqueous solution) | Brown precipitate | Presence of tannins |
| 4. HCHO/concentrated HCl (boiling, addition of ferric alum and $CH_3COONa$) | Blue color | Presence of hydrolysable tannins |
| 5. Mg/concentrated HCl test [Shinoda's test, carried out for an ethanolic solution of the dried material, the acid was added first, warmed to recognize changes in color then Mg was added] | Red color | Presence of flavonoids and/or their glycosides |

### 4.2.2. Chromatographic investigation

For the characterization and isolation of the phenolic constituents of the aerial parts extract, the following chromatographic investigations were carried out.

### 4.2.2.1. Paper chromatographic investigation and electrophoretic investigation

Two dimensional paper chromatography (2DPC) of the extract performed as described before (section E-1.1 in the previous chapter), revealed the presence of complicated phenolic spots. Corresponding spots gave positive response towards $FeCl_3$ spray reagent, some of which appeared under short UV light as dark purple spots which turned orange or lemon yellow when fumed with ammonia vapour or when sprayed with Naturstoff spray reagent, a typical character of flavone or flavonol derivatives (Harborne, 1982). Some spots have shown positive nitrous acid response indicative of ellagitannins other spots showed positive response with $KIO_3$ specific for galloyl esters (Haddock et al., 1982). Besides, paper electrophoretic analysis of the aqueous methanolic aerial parts extract proved the presence of ionic phenolic conjugates (positive $FeCl_3$ test, and mobility of the corresponding spots on the electrophoretic chromatogram).

For the isolation and structure elucidation of the phenolics contained in the extract, Sephadex column chromatography was then engaged.

### 4.2.2.2. Column chromatographic investigation

#### Fractionation of the extract

A portion of the aqueous EtOH extract thus obtained, was applied (**90** g dissolved in 100 ml bidistilled water) over Sephadex LH-20 (850 g) column (100 X 5 cm) and elution with methanol/bidistilled water mixtures of decreasing polarities for gradient elution led to the desorption of 12 individual fractions. The fractions dried, individually, in vacuum were tested for phenolics (Table 5) and then subjected to two dimensional paper chromatographic investigation (2DPC).

## Table (5): Characteristics of the column fractions (I– XII) of the extract

| Fraction | Water/ Methanol | Weight (g) | Color with FeCl$_3$ | Result with Mg/HCl | Characters |
|---|---|---|---|---|---|
| I | Water | 23.62 | No color | Negative | Sticky dark brown material of non phenolic characters. |
| I-1 | Water | 2.30 | Deep Blue | Negative | Buff amorphous powder of phenolic nature. |
| II | Water | 1.66 | Brown Green | Deep red | Light Brown powder of flavonoid nature. |
| III | 90:10 | 1.70 | Brown Green | Deep red | Brown material of flavonoid nature. |
| IV | 80:20 | 0.94 | Intense blue | Negative | Buff brown material of phenolic nature. |
| V | 70:30 | 1.95 | Intense blue | Negative | Buff amorphous powder of phenolic nature. |
| VI | 60:40 | 6.57 | Green | Deep Red | Light Brown powder of flavonoid nature. |
| VII | 50:50 | 1.89 | Intense blue | Negative | Light brown amorphous material of phenolic nature. |
| VIII | 40:60 | 1.58 | Intense blue | Negative | Light brown amorphous material of phenolic natur |

| Fraction | Water/ Methanol | Weight (gm) | Color with FeCl₃ | Result with Mg/HCl | Characters |
|---|---|---|---|---|---|
| IX | 30:70 | 2.50 | Intense blue | Negative | Amorphous material of phenolic nature. |
| X | 20:80 | 5.70 | Deep green | Deep red | Light yellow amorphous powder of flavonoid nature. |
| XI | 10:90 | 6.65 | Intense blue | Negative | Pale yellow amorphous powder of phenolic nature. |
| XII | Methanol | 4.25 | Brown | Negative | Pale yellow amorphous powder of phenolic nature. |
| lost | | 28.64 | | | |

### 4.3. Isolation of compounds (1-20) from the column fractions (I- XII)
### 4.4. Paper chromatographic analysis of fractions (I- XII)

Each of the collected 12 column fractions (I– XII), (Table 5) was subjected to 2DPC investigation, whereby chromogenic spray reagents specific for both phenolics and flavonoids (section B-7 in the previous chapter) were generally used. Based on the obtained results, each of the collected fractions (I- XII) was individually dealt with to isolate pure samples of the contained phenolics whenever possible.

**Fraction I**

2DPC of the material of this fraction showed that it is a non-phenolic material.

## Fraction I-1

Among the several minor constituents, which were shown under UV light on 2DPC of this fraction, one component compound **1** was found predominant. It appeared as blue coloured spot. In addition, it showed a distinct migration of its spot upon performing electrophoresis.

## Isolation of compound (1):

Compound **1** (71 mg) was isolated pure from fraction I-1 (2.3 g, eluted with $H_2O$) by repeated precipitation (thrice) with acetone from a concentrated aqueous solution of this fraction (903 mg).

## Identification of compound (1): 3-Methoxygallic acid 5-sodium sulphate

Compound **1** appeared as a blue spot under short UV light on paper chromatogram (PC) of $R_f$ values (Table 6) which migrates a distance of 1.4 cm on electrophoretic chromatogram.

It gave a blue colour with $FeCl_3$ and red colour after heating with aniline/xylose, specific for carboxylic acids (Smith, 1976). It exhibited UV absorption maxima in methanol (Table 6). On mild acid hydrolysis (aqueous 0.1 N HCl at 100 $^0C$, 3 min.), it yielded gallic acid 3-methyl ether (CoPC, $^1$H-NMR and $^{13}$C-NMR) as the only released phenolic. The hydrolysate was found to be free from any sugar material (CoPC), but it gave a heavy white ppt. with aqueous $BaCl_2$, thus proving the presence of sulphate moiety in the molecule of **1**. Atomic absorption analysis confirmed that the $SO_4$ radical(s) exist in the molecule of 1 as sodium sulfate (S). On negative ESI-MS, it gave an [M-Na]$^-$ ion at m/z =263 corresponding to Mr =286 . These data led to the tentative identification of **1** as 3-methoxygallic acid mono-sodium sulphate.

For achieving the structure of **1**, NMR spectral analysis was then undertaken. The $^1$H-NMR (Fig. 5) and $^{13}$C-NMR (Fig. 6) spectra (DMSO-$d_6$, room temperature), lent a support to the above given view and finally confirmed the structure of compound **1** as 3-methoxygallic acid 5-sodium sulphate, isolated previously from *Tamarix amplexicaulis* (Souleman *et al.*, 1998).

**Compound (1): 3-Methoxygallic acid 5-sodium sulphate**

**Table (6): Chromatographic and spectral data of compound (1)**

| 1. $R_f$ values (x 100) | 96 (H2O), 84(HOAc-6), 49 (BAW) |
|---|---|
| 2. UV spectral data $\lambda_{max}$ (nm), MeOH | 267, 297** |
| 3. Electrophoresis mobility | 1.4 cm |
| 4. $^1$H- NMR spectral data (DMSO-$d_6$)δ (ppm) | δ7.55 (1H, d, $J$=2 Hz, H-2), 7.24 (1H, d, $J$=2 Hz, H-6), 3.79 (3H, s, -OCH3) |
| 5. $^{13}$C-NMR spectral data (DMSO-$d_6$)δ (ppm) | 119.6 (C-1), 108.6 (C-2), 148.5 (C-3), 141.1 (C-4), 143.5(C-5), 117.3(C-6), 167.6 (C=O), 56.3 (OMe) |

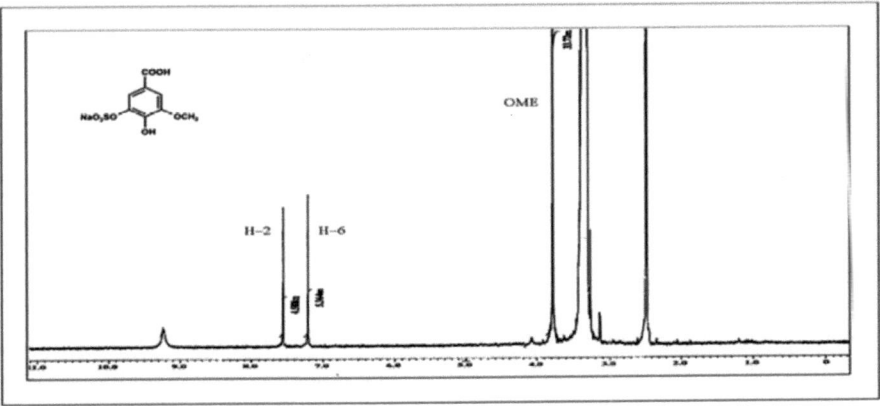

Fig. (5): $^1$H-NMR spectrum of compound

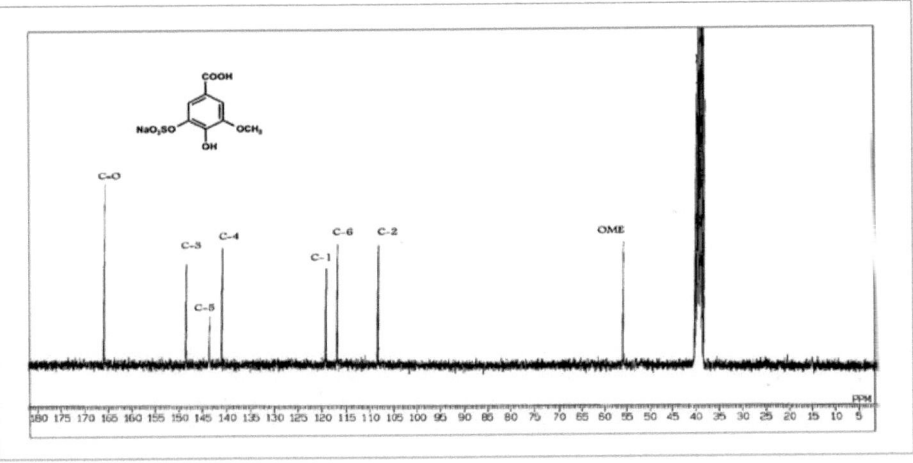

Fig. (6): $^{13}$C-NMR spectrum of compound (1)

## Fraction II

2DPC of fraction II showed one predominant component (compound 2) appearing as a blue coloured spot on PC under UV light. In addition, it showed a distinct migration of its spot upon performing electrophoresis.

## Isolation of compound (2)

Compound **2** (85 mg) was obtained pure by fractionation of 1.2 g of fraction II (1.66 g, eluted with water) over Sephadex LH-20 (17 g) column (30 x 2 cm) and elution with water.

## Identification of compound (2): Kaempferide 3, 7-disodium sulphate

Compound **2** (85 mg) was isolated as an off-white amorphous powder which exhibited chromatographic and anionic character on electrophoretic analysis similar to those of anionic flavonol (Barron et al., 1988). UV absorption maxima in MeOH (Table 6) and after addition of diagnostic shift reagents (Harborne and Williams, 1975) showed no shift with NaOAc or with NaOAc/$H_3BO_3$, a small shift with NaOMe and 28 nm shift with HCl. These data were consistent with 3, 7, 4'-trisubstituted kaempferol structure. On mild acid hydrolysis (0.1 N aq. HCl at 100 $^0$C for 3 mins) **2** yielded two intermediates **2a** (major, yellow spot on PC under UV light) and and **2b** (minor, dark purple spot on PC under UV light). The aqueous acidic hydrolysate gives a white ppt. with aq. $BaCl_2$ to prove the presence of $SO_4$ group. Atomic absorption analysis confirmed that the $SO_4$ radical(s) exist in the molecule of **2** as sodium sulphate. Intermediates **2a** and **2b** were individually separated by preparative paper chromatography. Their chromatographic, electrophoretic properties, UV absorption and $^1$H NMR spectral data proved a 7, 4'-disubstituted kaempferol structure for **2a** and a kaempferol 3, 4'- disubstituted structure for **2b**. Complete hydrolysis of the parent compound **2** (0.1 N aq. HCl at 100 C for 15 mins) yielded kaempferol 4'-methyl ether, kaempheride (CoPC, UV, EIMS, $^1$H and $^{13}$C NMR) and sodium sulphate ($BaCl_2$ test and atomic absorption analysis), a result which when incorporated with the above given analytical data proved the identity of **2a** as kaempferide 7-$OSO_3$Na and that of **2b** as kaempferide 3-$OSO_3$Na. Consequently, compound **2** is suggested to be kaempheride 3, 7-di-sodium sulphate. The parent compound **2** exhibited a molecular mass of 504 as indicated by ESI-MS analysis. The spectrum exhibited ions at $m/z$ 480 [M – Na - H]$^-$, 423 [M - $SO_3$ - H]$^-$ and 343 [M - $2SO_3$ - H]$^-$, corresponding to a molecular weight 504 and a molecular formula $C_{16}H_{10}O_{12}Na_2S_2$, as was confirmed by HRESIMS, m/z: 480.3569 [M − Na − H]⁻, (calc.: 480.3580). This and the above given data proved that **2** is kaempferide 3, 7-di-sodium sulphate. Further support for this view was obtained through NMR spectral analysis. The $^1H$ spectrum of **2** revealed in the aromatic region a pattern of signals though similar to that of the aglycone, keampferide, yet a distinction could be made through the recognition of the downfield shift of the proton signals of H − 6 and H − 8 (δ ppm 6.45 and 6.81, respectively), in comparison with the signal at δ ppm 6.20 and 6.45 of the corresponding protons in the spectrum of the free aglycone. This is obviously due to sulphation at position 7 of the kaempferide moiety. From the $^{13}C$ spectrum of (**2**) the recognized up field shift (Δ δ = 3.1 ppm) of the resonance of C-3 and the accompanying downfield shift ( Δ δ =9.8 ppm and Δ δ = 2.3 ppm) of the signals of carbons C-2 and C4, respectively, all in comparison with the chemical shift of the corresponding signal in the spectrum of the aglycone are attributed to sulphation at C-3 of the aglycone moiety. Similar set of shifts was recognized due to sulphation at C-7. Such shifts are well known from the work (Nawwar and Buddrus, 1981). Other resonances in this spectrum exhibited chemical shift values which were in close agreement to the achieved structure of compound (**2**) as kaempferide 3,7-di-sodium sulphate, a natural product which represents to the best of our knowledge a new natural product.

**Compound 2: Kaempferide 3, 7-disodium sulphate**

## Table (7): Chromatographic and spectral data of compounds (2, 2a and 2b)

|  | Compound 2 |
|---|---|
| 1. $R_f$ values (x 100) | 0.85($H_2O$), 0.73 (HOAc-6), 0.25 (BAW) |
| 2. UV Spectral Data $\lambda_{max}$ (nm), MeOH | MeOH: 265, 300 shoulder, 342; NaOMe: 270, 380; NaOAc: 264, 310,342; NaOAc-$H_3BO_3$: 266, 300 shoulder, 340; $AlCl_3$: 270, 302, 345, 380 (shoulder); HCl (30 mins): 270, 370. |
| 3. Electrophoresis mobility | 5.6 cm |
| 4. ESIMS (negative mode), $m/z$: | $m/z$ 480 [M – Na - H]⁻, 423 [M - $SO_3$ - H]⁻ and 343 [M - $2SO_3$ - H] |
| HRESIMS, $m/z$: | 480.3569 [M – Na – H]⁻, (calc.: 480.3580). |
| 5. $^1$H- NMR spectral data (DMSO-$d_6$)δ (ppm) | 8.19 (2H, $d$, $J$ = 8.5 Hz, H-2' and H-6'), 7.1 (2H, $d$, $J$=8.5 Hz, H-3' and H-5'), 6.82 (IH, $d$, $J$=2 Hz, H-8); 6.45 (1H, $d$, $J$=2 Hz, H-6). |
| 6. $^{13}$C-NMR spectral data (DMSO-$d_6$)δ (ppm) | 156.5 (C-2), 132.6 (C-3), 178.2 (C-4), 160.0 (C-5), 101.6 (C-6), 159.8 (C-7), 98.8 (C-8), 155.3 (C-9), 105.9 (C-10), 121.2 (C-1'), 129.8 (C-2' & C-6'), 114.4 (C-3' & C-5'), 160.6 (C-4'), 56.3 (C-4'OMe). Mild Acid hydrolysis (30 mg in 10 ml aqueous methanol, 1:1, of 0.1 N aq. HCl at 100 C for 3 mins) of **2a and 2b**. |

|  | Compound 2a |
|---|---|
| 1. $R_f$ values (x 100) | 0.45 ($H_2O$), 0.40 (HOAc-6), 0.26 (BAW) |
| 2. UV spectral data $\lambda$max (nm), MeOH | MeOH: 265, 365; NaOMe: 263, 389; NaOAc: 264, 310, 364; NaOAc-$H_3BO_3$: 265, 300 shoulder, 360; $AlCl_3$: 270, 302, 345, 400 shoulder; HCl: 270, 368. |
| 3. Electrophoresis mobility | 2.5 cm |
| 4. $^1H$- NMR spectral data (DMSO-$d_6$) $\delta$ (ppm) | 8.11 (2H, $d$, $J$ = 8.5 Hz, H-2' and H-6'), 7.03 (2H, $d$, $J$=8.5 Hz, H-3' and H-5'), 6.78 (1H, $d$, $J$=2 Hz, H-8); 6.40 (1H, $d$, $J$=2 Hz, H-6). |
| 1. $R_f$ values (x 100) | Compound 2b |
|  | 0.48 ($H_2O$), 0.42 (HOAc), 0.30 (BAW) |
| 2. UV spectral data $\lambda$max (nm), MeOH | MeOH: 267, 342; NaOMe: 270, 350 decomposion; NaOAc: 269, 310, 346; NaOAc-$H_3BO_3$: 267, 342; AlCl3: 270, 304, 345, 400 shoulder; HCl: 270, 367 |
| 3. Electrophoresis mobility | 3 cm |
| 4. $^1H$- NMR spectral data (DMSO-$d_6$) $\delta$ (ppm) | 8.10 (2H, $d$, $J$ = 8.5 Hz, H-2' and H-6'), 7.15 (2H, $d$, $J$=8.5 Hz, H-3' and H-5'), 6.43 (1H, $d$, $J$=2 Hz, H-8), 6.21 (1H, $d$, $J$=2 Hz, H-6). |
| 1. $R_f$ values (x 100) 2. UV spectral data $\lambda$max (nm), MeOH | Kaempferide aglycone: 0.92 (BAW) |

| | |
|---|---|
| | MeOH: 267, 300 shoulder, 367; NaOMe: 280, 404; NaOAc: 272, 310, 384; NaOAc-$H_3BO_3$: 267, 300 shoulder, 364; $AlCl_3$: 270, 304, 345, 420 shoulder; 367. |
| 3. $^1$H- NMR spectral data (DMSO-d6)δ (ppm) | 8.15 (2H, d, J = 8.5 Hz, H-2' and H-6'), 7.05 (2H, d, J=8.5 Hz, H-3' and H-5'), 6.45 (IH, d, J=2 Hz, H-8); 6.20 (1H, d, J=2 Hz, H-6). |
| 4. $^{13}$C-NMR spectral data (DMSO-d6)δ (ppm) | 146.7 (C-2), 135.7 (C-3), 175.9 (C-4), 160.7 (C-5), 98.2 (C-6), 163.9 (C-7), 93.5 (C-8), 156.2 (C-9), 103.0 (C-10), 123.2 (C-1'), 121.3 (C-1'), 129.5 (C-2' & C-6'), 114.2 (C-3' & C-5'), 160.2 (C-4'), 55.9 (C-4'OMe) |

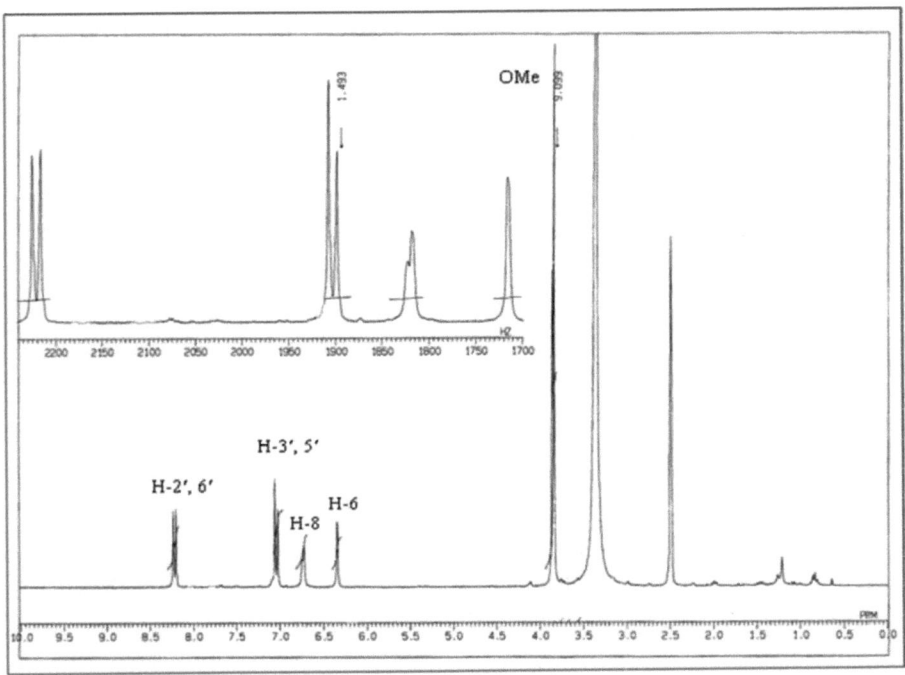

Fig. (7): $^1$H –NMR spectrum of compound (2)

## Fraction III

Among the several minor constituents which were shown under UV light on 2DPC of this fraction, two components were found as major spots **3**, **4** and appeared as blue coloured spot. Both showed a distinct migration of its spot upon performing electrophoresis.

## Isolation of compounds 3 and 4

Compounds **3** and **4** were individually isolated pure (112 mg and 96 mg, respectively) through repeated preparative PC of the material of fraction III (1.70 g, eluted with 10 % MeOH), using water as solvent.

## Identification of compound (3): Kaempferide 3- sodium sulphate

Compound **3** (112 mg) was isolated as an off-white amorphous powder which exhibited chromatographic and anionic character on electrophoretic analysis similar to those of anionic flavonol (Barron *et al.*, 1988). Compound (**3**) appeared as a dark purple spot on PC under UV light, which changed to lemon yellow on exposure to ammonia vapors, and to yellow when sprayed with Naturstoff reagent. Complete hydrolysis of (**3**) (8 mg in 5 ml, 0.1 N aq. HCl, at 100° C for 15 minutes) yielded Kaempferol 4'-methyl ether, Kaempferide (4 mg) which was filtered on from the cooled hydrolysate. The $R_f$-values, UV, $^1$H and $^{13}$C-NMR spectral analysis data of this aglycone are identical with those of compound (**17\***) described on (Table 21) (Fig. 46 & 47). The aqueous acidic hydrolysate gave a white ppt. with aq. $BaCl_2$ to prove the presence of $SO_4$ radical. Atomic absorption analysis confirmed that the $SO_4$ radical exists in the molecule of **3** as sodium sulphate. The chromatographic, electrophoretic properties, UV absorption and $^1$H- NMR data proved a kaempferol 3, 4'-disubstituted structure for **3** (Fig. 8) (Table 8). Substitution at the C–3 of the aglycone was obvious from the dark purple coloration of the spot of **3** on PC, in addition, the chemical shifts of H-6 and H-8 are resonating at δppm closely similar to those reported to the aglycone, kaempferol. Finally, compound (**3**) is identified as kaempferide 3-$OSO_3Na$ (Tomas-Barberan *et al.*, 1990).

**Compound (3): Kaempferide 3- OSO3Na (3)**

**Table (8): Chromatographic and spectral data of compound (3)**

| | | |
|---|---|---|
| 1. | $R_f$ values (x 100) | 0.48 ($H_2O$), 0.42 (HOAc-6), 0,30 (BAW 3 cm |
| 2. | Electrophoretic mobility | |
| 3. | UV Spectral Data $\lambda_{max}$ (nm), MeOH | MeOH: 267, 342; <br> NaOMe: 270, 350 decomposion; <br> NaOAc: 269, 310, 346; <br> NaOAc-$H_3BO_3$: 267, 342; <br> AlCl3: 270, 304, 345, 400 shoulder; <br> HCl: 270, 367 |
| 4. | $^1$H- NMR Spectral Data($CD_3$)$_2$CO or (DMSO-$d_6$) δ (ppm) | 8.10 (2H, d, J = 8.5 Hz, H-2' and H-6'), <br> 7.15 (2H, d, J=8.5 Hz, H-3' and H-5'), <br> 6.43 (1H, d,J=2 Hz 2H, H-8), <br> 6.21 (IH, d, J=2 Hz, H-6). |

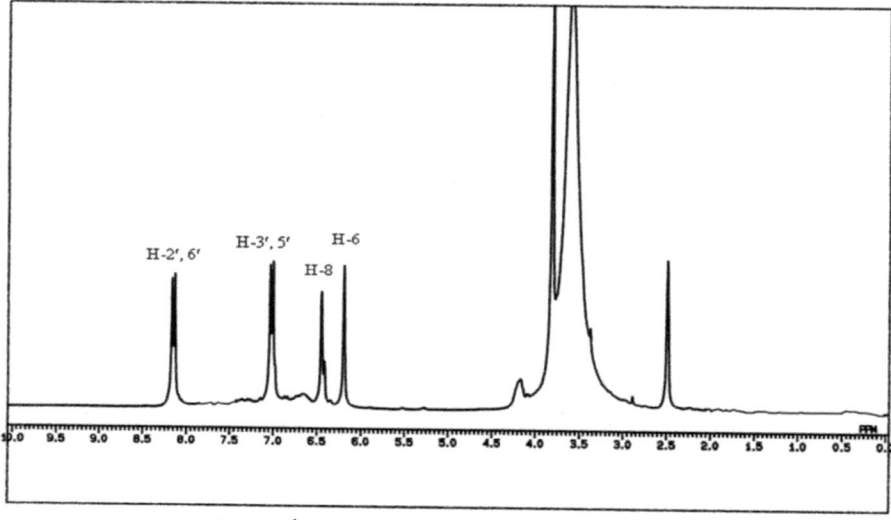

Fig. (8): $^1$H –NMR spectrum of compound (3)

## Identification of compound (4): Tamarexitin 3- sodium sulphate

Compound **4** was isolated as an off-white amorphous powder (96 mg) which exhibited chromatographic (dark purple spot on PC turning dull yellow when fumed with ammonia, dull yellow when sprayed with Natur-Stuff) and anionic character on electrophoretic analysis similar to those exhibited by anionic flavonols (Barron *et al.*, 1988a; b; El-Mousallamy *et al.*, 2000; Souleman *et al.*, 1998), (Table 9).

Complete hydrolysis of (**4**) (14 mg in 5 ml, 0.1 N aq. HCl, at 100°C for 15 minutes) yielded quercetin 4'-methyl ether, tamarixetin (5 mg) which was filtered on from the cooled hydrolysate. The $R_f$-values, UV, $^1H$ and $^{13}C$-NMR of this aglycone are identical with those of compound (18) described on (Table 22) (Fig. 48 &49). The aqueous acidic hydrolysate gave a white ppt. with aq. $BaCl_2$ to prove the presence of $SO_4$ group. Atomic absorption analysis confirmed that the $SO_4$ radical exists in the molecule of **4** as sodium sulphate. The chromatographic, electrophoretic properties, UV absorption, $^1H$ and $^{13}C$-NMR data of compound **4** proved a 3, 4'- disubstituted quercetin structure (Table 9) (Fig. 9&10). Substitution at the C–3 of the aglycone was quite obvious from the dark purple coloration of the spot of **4** on PC. Finally, compound **4** is identified as tamarexitin 3-$OSO_3Na$. (Tomas-Barberan *et al.*, 1990).

**Compound (4): Tamarexitin 3-$OSO_3Na$**

## Table (9): Chromatographic and spectral data of compound (4)

| | |
|---|---|
| 1. $R_f$ values (x 100) | 54 ($H_2O$), 45 (HOAc-6), 56 (BAW) |
| 2. UV Spectral Data $\lambda_{max}$ (nm), MeOH | MeOH: 252 inf., 267, 343;<br>NaOMe: 269, 320, 389;<br>NaOAC: 255 inf., 272, 388;<br>NaOAc + $H_3BO_3$: 254, 267, 345;<br>$AlCl_3$: 268, 274, 300, 412;<br>$AlCl_3$ + HCl: 254, 268, 390. |
| 3. Electrophoretic mobility (cm) | 2.7 cm |
| 4. $^1$H- NMR Spectral Data ($CD_3(2)CO$) or (DMSO-$d_6$) δ (ppm) | 6.20 (1H, $d$, $J$ =2 Hz, H-6),<br>6.40 (1H, $d$, $J$ = 2 Hz, H-8),<br>7.10 (1H, $d$, $J$ = 8 Hz, H-5'),<br>7.62 (m, H-2' and H-6'), 3.83 (s, Me-4'). |
| 5. $^{13}$C-NMR Spectral Data (DMSO-$d_6$)δ (ppm) | 156.64 (C – 2), 132.63 (C – 3), 177.38 (C – 4), 161.22 (C – 5), 99.58 (C – 6), 166.89 (C – 7), 94.02 (C – 8), 156.98 (C – 9), 103.34 (C – 10), 123.03 (C – 1'), 115.52 (C - 2'), 146.12 (C – 3'), 150.09 (C – 4'), 111.58 (C – 5'), 121.15 (C – 6'), 55.65 ( Me-4'). |

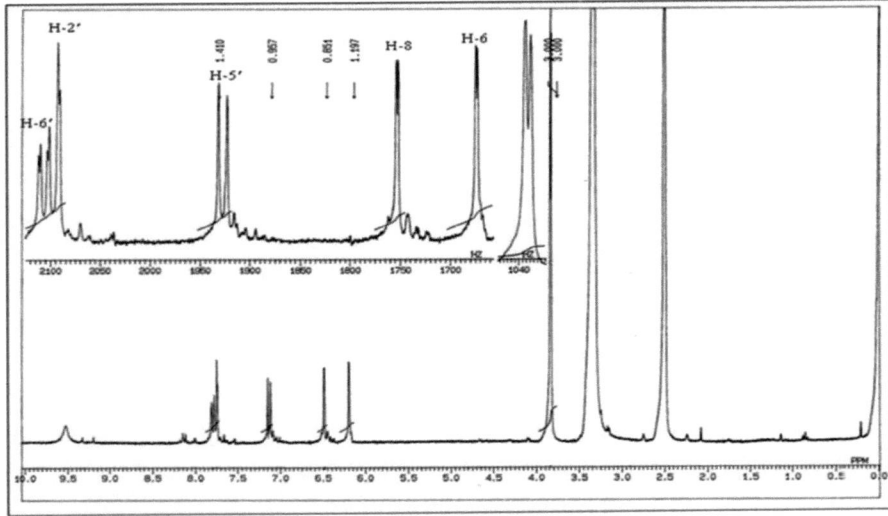

Fig. (9): $^1$H –NMR spectrum of compound (4)

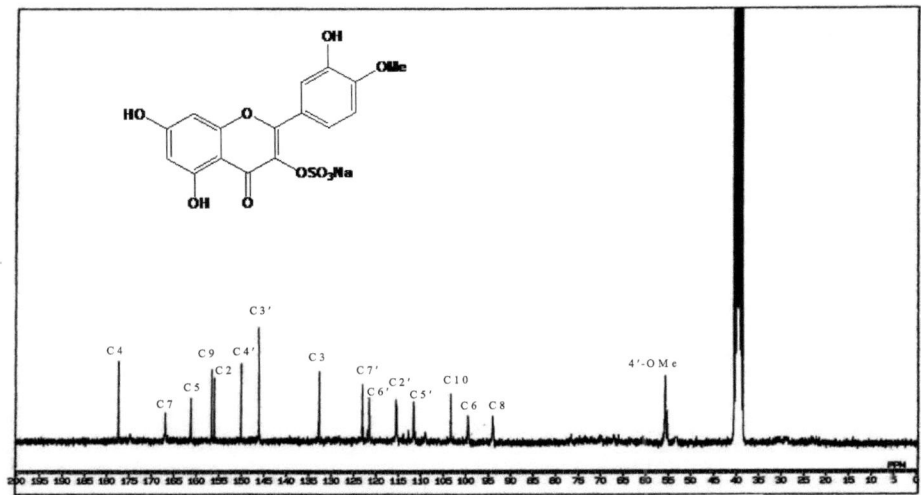

Fig. (10): $^{13}$C-NMR spectrum of compound (4)

## Fraction IV

This fraction showed two major spots on PC under short UV light, possessing phenolic acid nature (blue or brown colour with $FeCl_3$ and red color after heating with aniline/xylose, specific for carboxylic acid.

## Isolation of compounds (5) and (6):

Each of compounds 5 and 6 were separated pure (41 mg and 43 mg, respectively) from 240 mg of fraction IV (940 mg, eluted with 20 % MeOH) by applying Sephadex LH-20 column(12 g, 30 x 2 cm) fractionation and elution with *n*-BuOH water saturated.

## Identification of compound (5): Gallic acid

2DPC showed compound 5 (41 mg) as a blue spot under short UV light of $R_f$ values (Table 10) which gave a blue colour with $FeCl_3$ and red color after heating with aniline/xylose spray reagent specific for carboxylic acid (Smith, 1976). It exhibited UV absorption maxima in methanol (Table 10) and on negative ESI-MS, it gave an [M-H]⁻ ion at $m/z = 169$ (Fig. 11). These data led to the tentative identification of 5 as 3, 4, 5-trihydroxybenzoic acid, gallic acid (Nawwar *et al.*, 1984e).

For confirming the structure of 5, NMR spectral analysis was then undertaken, the ¹H-NMR spectrum (DMSO-$d_6$, room temperature), lent a support to the above given view and revealed only one singlet in the aromatic region at δ 6.98 ppm (Table 10), assignable to the two equivalent H-2 and H-6 protons of the symmetrical gallic acid molecule. The ¹³C-NMR spectra (Fig.12) finally confirmed the achieved structure of 5 and revealed five distinct $sp^2$ carbon resonances corresponding to the seven carbons (Table 10) with chemical shift values identical with those reported for gallic acid (Nawwar *et al.*, 1984).

**Compound (5): Gallic acid**

**Table (10): Chromatographic and spectral data of compound (5)**

| 1. | $R_f$ values (x 100) | 44 ($H_2O$), 55 (HOAc-6), 72 (BAW) |
|---|---|---|
| 2. | UV spectral data $\lambda_{max}$ (nm), MeOH | 272 |
| 3. | $^1$H-NMR spectra data (DMSO-$d_6$)δ (ppm) | 6.98 (2H, s, H-2 and H-6) |
| 4. | $^{13}$C-NMR spectral data (DMSO-$d_6$)δ (ppm) | 120.6 (C-1), 108.8 (C-2 and C-6), 145.5 (C-3 and C-5), 138.1 (C-4), 167.7 (C=O) |

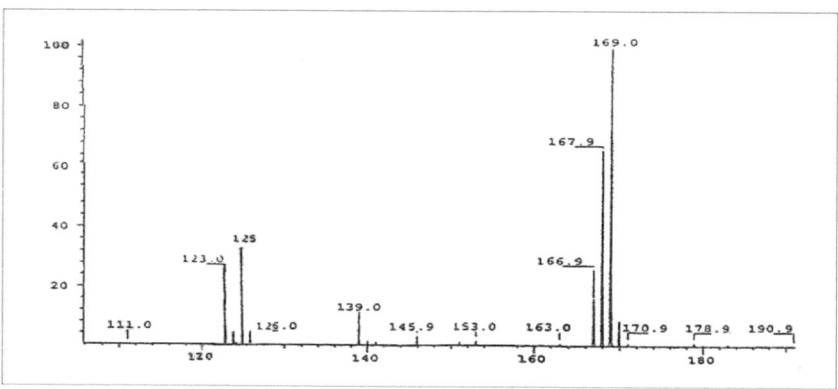

Fig. (11): ESI-MS spectrum of compound (5)

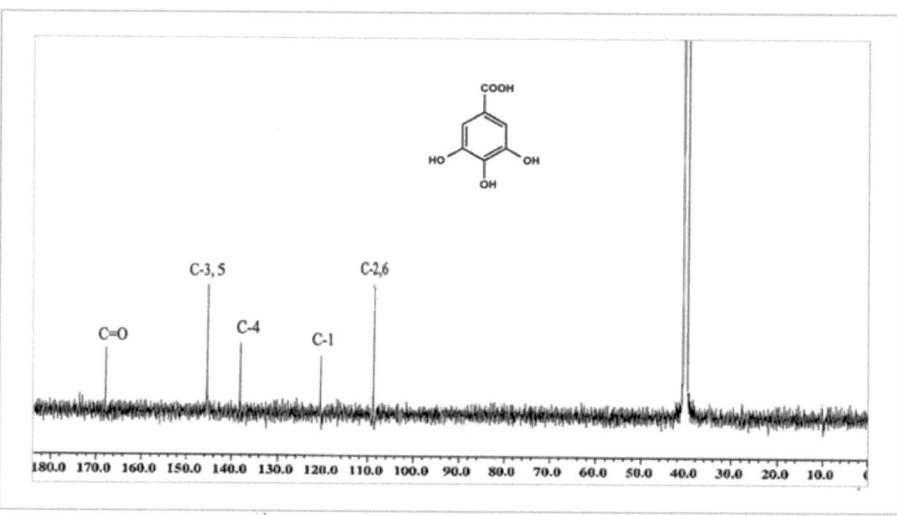

Fig. (12): $^{13}$C-NMR spectrum of compound (5)

## Identification of compound (6): 3-Methoxygallic acid

Compound **6** (43 mg) was isolated as an amorphous off white powder. It appeared on paper chromatograms as blue spot under short UV light of $R_f$ values (Table11). Its spot on 2DPC gave a blue colour with FeCl3 and red colour after heating with aniline/xylose, specific for carboxylic acid (Smith, 1976). On mild acid hydrolysis (aqueous 0.1 N HCl at 100 $^0$C, 3 min.), it was recovered unchanged. It exhibited UV absorption maxima in methanol (Table11) and on negative ESI-MS, it gave an [M-H]- ion at m/z = 183 (Fig.13). These data led to the tentative identification of 6 as a methoxy gallic acid.

For confirming the structure of **6** and specifying the site of attachment of the methoxy group NMR spectral analysis was then undertaken, the $^1$H-NMR (Table 11) and $^{13}$C-NMR spectrum (Fig. 14 and Table 11) (DMSO-d$_6$, room temperature), lent a support to the above given view and finally confirmed the structure of compound **6** as 3-methoxygallic acid (El-Mousallamy *et al.*, 2000).

**Compound (6): 3-Methoxygallic acid**

## Table (11): Chromatographic and spectral data of compound (6)

| | | |
|---|---|---|
| 1. | $R_f$ values (x 100) | 50 ($H_2O$), 53 (HOAc-15), 84(BAW) |
| 2. | UV spectral data $\lambda$max (nm), MeOH | 273 |
| 3. | $^1$H- NMR spectral data (DMSO-$d_6$)$\delta$ (ppm) | 7.24 (1H, d, J=2.5 Hz, H-2)<br>7.15 (1H, d, J=2.5 Hz, H-6)<br>3.8 (s, 3H, 3-OMe) |
| 4. | $^{13}$C-NMR spectral data (DMSO-$d_6$)$\delta$ (ppm) | 120.9 (C-1), 105.2 (C-2), 148.6 (C-3), 139.5 (C-4), 145.9 (C-5), 111.26 (C-6), 167.3 (C=O), 56.3 (3-OMe) |

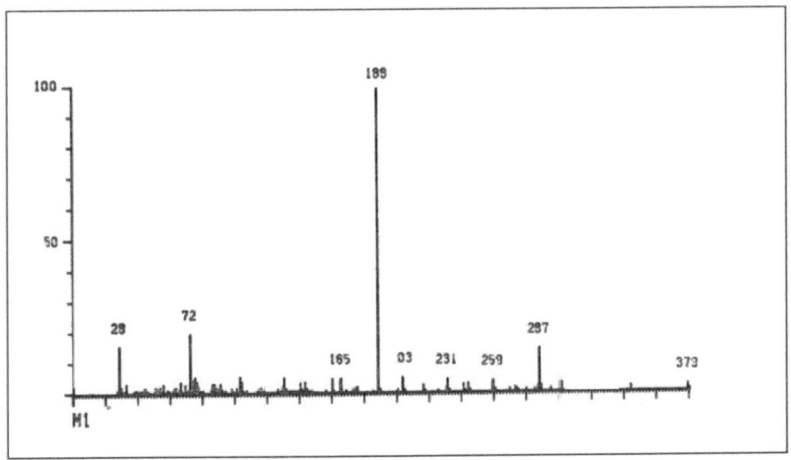

Fig. (13): Negative ESI-MS of compound (6)

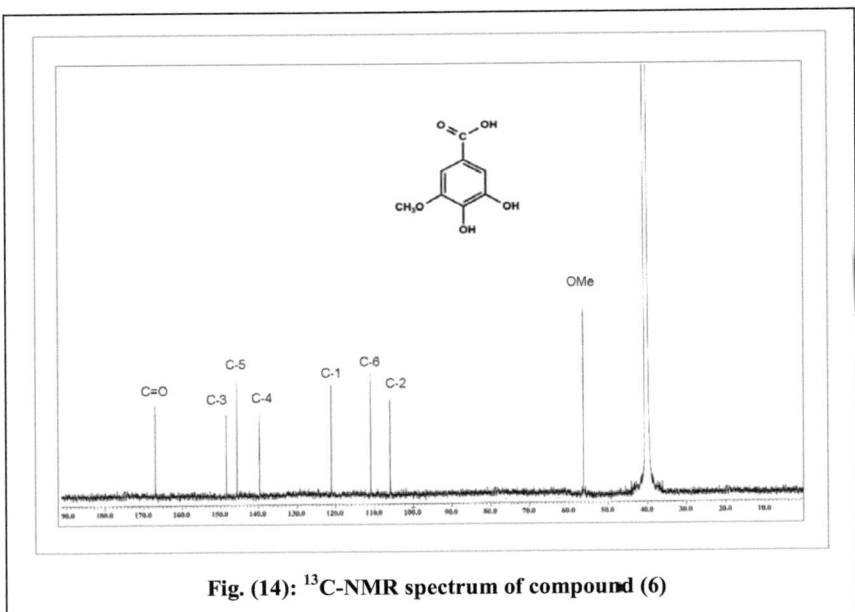

Fig. (14): $^{13}$C-NMR spectrum of compound (6)

## Fraction V

2DPC of this fraction revealed the presence of polyphenolic component that was found to possess the properties of galloyl esters (pink colour with saturated aqueous $KIO_3$ and intense blue colour with $FeCl_3$ spray reagents).

## Isolation of compound (7):

Polyamide column (25 g, 45 x 2.5 cm) fractionation of 880 mg amount of fraction V (1.95 g, eluted with 30 % MeOH) and elution with 30 % aqueous MeOH yielded pure samples of 7 (49 mg).

## Identification of compound (7): 2, 3-di-*O*-Galloyl-(α/β)-$^4C_1$-glucopyranose

Compound 7 (45 mg) gave a blue colour with $FeCl_3$, and a pink color with $KIO_3$ on PC indicative of gallotannins. It possessed $R_f$-values, UV spectral data (Table 12) and negative ESI-MS spectrum (Fig. 15) showing [M-H]$^-$ ion peak at 483 corresponding to Mr = 484, identical with those reported for digalloyl glucoses (Nawwar *et al.*, 1984c).

Complete acid hydrolysis of compound 7, yielded gallic acid (CoPC, UV spectral data, $^1$H-NMR analysis) and glucose (CoPC), while on controlled acid hydrolysis it yielded only, one intermediate 7a, which was separated by PPC, using BAW as solvent. 7a was then subjected to chromatographic, UV-spectral and negative ESI-MS (Fig. 16) analysis, which proved its identity as monogalloyl glucose. The site of attachment of the two galloyl moieties in the molecule of 7 were then determined through $^1$H- (Fig. 17) and $^{13}$C-NMR analyses (Fig. 18) which gave similar data (Table 12) to those reported previously for 2,3-di-*O*-galloyl-(α/β)-$^4C_1$-glucopyranose or nilocitin (Nawwar *et al.*, 1984).

Compound (7): 2, 3-di-*O*-Galloyl-(α/β)-$^4C_1$-glucopyranose

## Table (12): Chromatographic and spectral data of compound (7)

| | |
|---|---|
| 1. $R_f$ values (x 100) | 69 $H_2O$, 74 HOAc, 33 BAW |
| 2. UV spectral data $\lambda_{max}$ (nm) | 276 |
| 3. $^1$H-NMR spectral data (DMSO-$d_6$)δ (ppm) | α-glucouse<br>5.4 (1H, *d*, *J*=3.3 Hz, H-1)<br>4.92 (1H, *dd*, *J*=8 & 3.3 Hz, H-2)<br>5.78 (1H, *t*,*J*=8 Hz, H-3)<br>3.1-4.0 (*m*, H-4,5,6)<br><br>β-glucouse<br>4.98 (1H, *d*, *J*=7.5 Hz, H-1)<br>5.08 (1H, *t*, *J*=7.5Hz, H-2)<br>5.41(1H, *t*, *J*=7.5Hz, H-3)<br>3.1-4.0(*m*, H-4,5,6)<br><br>Galloyl in α- and β- anomers<br>6.87(2H,*s*), 6.81(4H,*s*), 6.79(2H, *s*) |
| 4. $^{13}$C-NMR spectral data (DMSO-$d_6$)δ (ppm) | α-Glucose<br>89.3 (C-1), 72.2 (C-2), 72.2 (C-3), 68.3 (C-4), 72.2 (C-5), 60.6 (C-6)<br><br>β-Glucose<br>94.5 (C-1), 73.1 (C-2), 75.5 (C-3), 68.3 (C-4), 76.7(C-5), 60.6(C-6)<br><br>Galloyl in α- and β- anomers<br>120.64,121.38,121.42 (C-1' α/β',1" α/β ), 109.97 (C-2',6' α/β, 2",6" α/β), 145.64 (C-3',5' α/β,3",5" α/β), 138.67,138.9 (C-4' α/β,4" α/β), 164.8,165.2,165.4,165.5 (C=O α/β, C'=O α/β) |

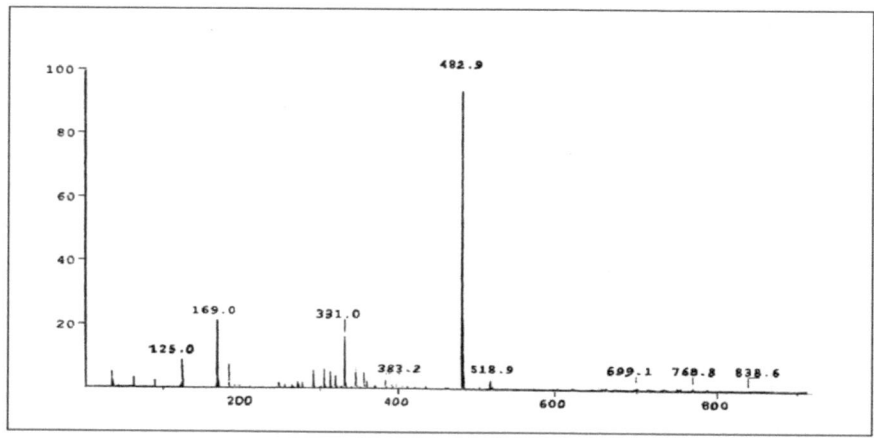

Fig. (15): Negative ESI-MS spectrum of compound (7)

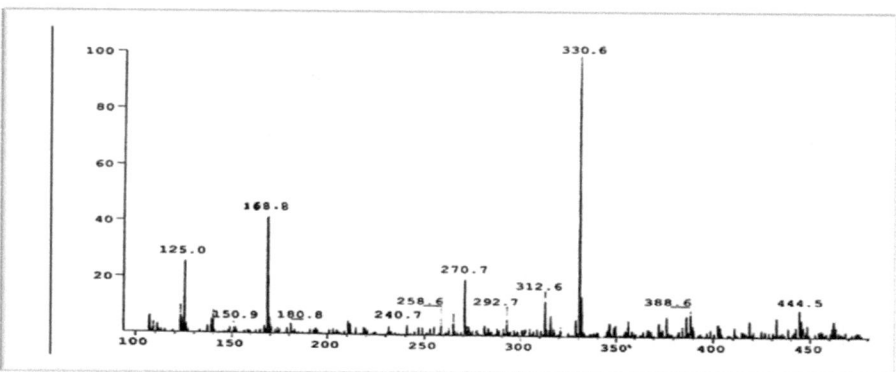

Fig. (16): Negative ESI-MS spectrum of compound (7a)

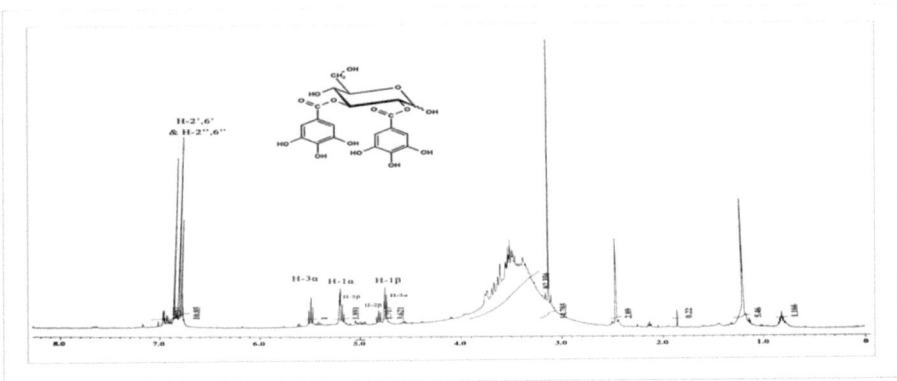

Fig. (17): $^1$H-NMR spectrum of compound (7)

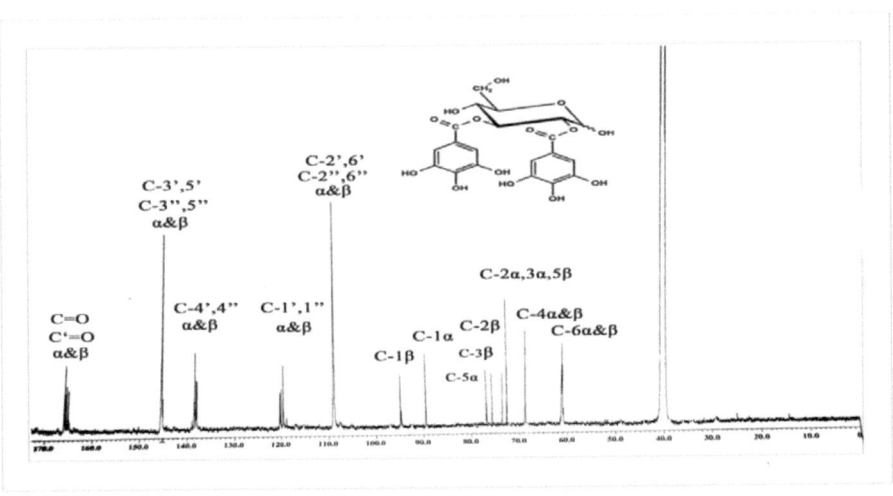

Fig (18): $^{13}$C-NMR spectrum of compound (7)

## Fraction VI

The brown amorphous material of this fraction showed three major phenolic spots (brown green colour with $FeCl_3$ spray reagent) with flavonoid characters which appeared on chromatogram under UV light as dark purple spots turning yellow on fuming with ammonia vapour and red color after heating with aniline/xylose, specific for carboxylic acid.

## Isolation of compounds 8, 9 and 10

Compounds **8**, **9** and **10** were individually isolated pure (58 mg, 40 mg and 29 mg, respectively) from fraction VI (6.57 g, eluted with 40 % MeOH) by repeated Sephadex LH-20 (30 g) column (45 x 2.5 cm) fractionation of 2.6 g material of this fraction.

## Identification of compound (8): Quercetin 3-*O*-*β*-glucuronide (miquelianin)

The yellowish amorphous powder of compound **8** (58 mg) was found to possess the following chromatographic properties: dark purple spot on PC under UV light, which changed to orange upon $NH_3$ vapour exposure or spraying with Naturstoff. It turned green upon spraying with $FeCl_3$ and gave positive reaction with aniline / xylose spray specific for carboxylic acids (Harborne, 1973; Smith, 1976). Moderate migration in aqueous and organic solvents on PC is shown (Table **13**). The UV spectral characteristics in methanol and on addition of shift reagents of 8 (Table 13) were similar to those reported for quercetin 3-*O*-glucuronide (Moon *et al.*, 2001).

The $^1$H-NMR spectrum (Fig. 19) showed H -6 and H -8, with $J_{meta}$ = 2.4 Hz, and a pattern typical of a 1,2,4-trisubstituted hydoxylated benzene with δ 7.96 (d, $J_{meta}$ = 1.7 Hz, H-2'), 7.4 (1H, *dd*, *J* = 8.5 Hz and 1.7, H-6'), 6.81 (1H, d, *J*= 8.5 Hz, H-5'), corresponding to a quercetin aglycone, whereas the H-1"chemical shift was found at 5.3 ppm (*d*, *J* = 7 Hz), (Table 13) thus confirming that (8) is quercetin 3-*O*-glycoside (Smolarz *et al.*, 2002; Tatsis *et al.*, 2007). Furthermore, the structure of 8 was confirmed by $^{13}$C-NMR analysis (Fig. 20). In the received spectrum the glucuronic carbons resonance located at chemical shifts quite identical to those reported for the glucuronic moiety in flavonol 3-*O*-glucuronides (Nawwar *et al.*, 1984b). Consequently, compound **8** is identified as quercetin-3-*O*-*β*-$^4C_1$- glucuronide (Smolarz *et al.*, 2008; Yasukawa and Takido, 1987).

**Compound (8): Quercetin 3-$O$-β-$^4C_1$-glucuronide**

**Table (13): Chromatographic and spectral data of compound (8)**

| | | |
|---|---|---|
| 1. | $R_f$ – values (X100) | 67 ($H_2O$), 41 (6% HOAc) and 40 (BAW) |
| 2. | UV Spectral data λ $_{max}$ (nm) | MeOH: 254,361, NaOAc: 268,382<br>$H_3BO_3$: 272,299sh,379, $AlCl_3$: 274,303sh, 433,<br>NaOMe: 271,409 |
| 3. | $^1$H-NMR spectral data (DMSO-$d_6$) δ (ppm) | Quercetin moiety (Aglycone part):<br>6.09 (1H, $d$, $J$ = 2.4 Hz, H-6), 6.4 (1H, $d$, $J$ = 2.4 Hz, H-8), 7.96 (d, $J_{meta}$ = 1.7 Hz, H-2'), 6.81 (1H, $d$, $J$ = 8.5 Hz, H-5'), 7.4 (1H, $dd$, $J$ = 8.5 Hz and 1.7 Hz, H-6').<br>Glucuronic acid moiety (sugar part):<br>5.3 ($d$, $J$ = 7 Hz, H-1''), 3.2- 3.4 ($m$, sugar protons) |
| 4. | $^{13}$C-NMR Spectral Data (DMSO-$d_6$)δ (ppm | Quercetin: 157.75 (C-2), 132,02(C-3), 178.63(C-4), 162.40 (C-5), 99.59 (C-6), 165.43 (C-7), 94.59 (C-8), 157.75(C-9), 105,10 (C-10) , 122.92(C-1'), 116.97 (C-2'), 145.41 (C -3'), 149.32 (C-4' ), 115.61 (C-5'), 122.32 (C -6')<br>Glucuronic:<br>103.99 (C-1''), 71.6 (C-2''), 74.0 ( C -3''), 76.49 (C - 4''), 76.49 (C -5''), 169.7 (C - 6''). |

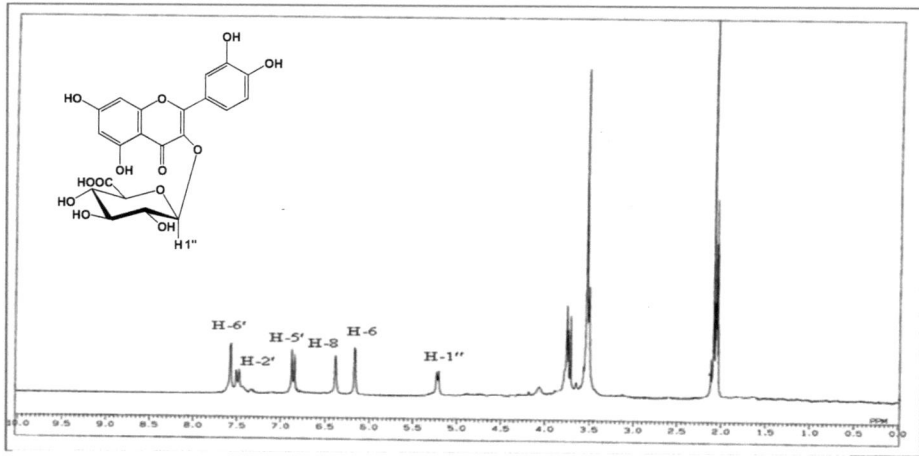

Fig. (19): $^1$H-NMR spectrum of compound (8)

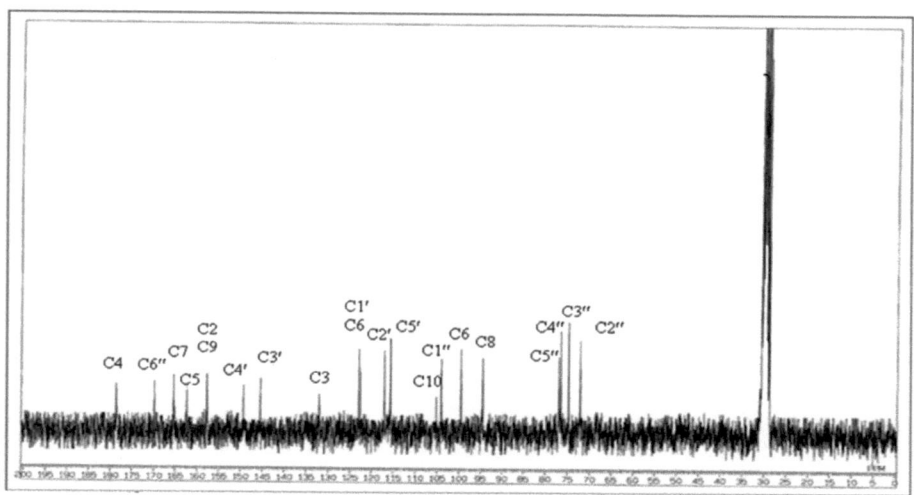

Fig. (20): $^{13}$C-NMR spectrum of compound (8)

## Identification of compound (9): Kaempferol 3- O-β-glucuronide

Compound (9) was isolated as a light brown amorphous powder (40 mg). It appeared as a dark purple on PC and turned yellow to orange upon exposure to ammonia vapors, under short UV light (254 nm). Compound (9) gave positive reaction with aniline / xylose spray reagent specific for carboxylic acids (Harborne, 1973; Smith, 1976) and showed $R_f$ = 40 (H$_2$O), 58 (6% Acetic acid), and 32 (BAW) (Table 14). Complete acid and enzymatic hydrolysis yielded kaempferol and glucuronic acid (CoPC).

The UV absorption data in methanol (Table 14) showed absorbance at 267nm representing band II and 353 nm for band I. Upon addition of sodium methoxide, a bathochromic shift occurred (49 nm) in band I and (8 nm) in band II indicating the presence of hydroxyl group at 4'. On addition of AlCl$_3$, bathochromic shift (55 nm) in band I indicating the presence of hydroxyl group at 5. On addition on HCL, no change occurred confirming the absence of orthodihydroxy groups. Presence of hydroxyl group free at position 7 allowed a bathochromic shift (8 nm) in band II upon addition of sodium acetate.

$^1$H-NMR spectral analysis of compound 9 (Fig.21), (DMSO-$d_6$, room temperature), confirmed a 3-*O*-substituted kaempferol structure due to the absence of appreciable shifts on the aromatic protons resonances on ring A which showed signals at δ ppm 6.74 (1H, broad *s*, H-8), 6.52 (1H, broad *s*, H-6). The identity of kaempferol was ascertained by the presence of signals at δ ppm 7.92 (2H, *d*, *J*= 8 Hz, H-2', H-6') and 6.94 (2H, *d*, *J*= 8 Hz, H-3', H-5'). The presence of a glucuronide moiety followed from the anomeric glucuronide acid proton signal at δppm 5.48 (1H, *d*, *J*= 7.5 Hz, H-1"), thus proving also β configuration of this moiety. Other signals of sugar protons appeared at 3.18-3.71 (*m*, sugar protons). Compound **9** was, therefore identified to be Kaempferol-3-*O*-β-D-glucuronide (Nawwar *et al.*, 1984b).

**Compound 9: Kaempferol-3-*O*-β-D-glucuronide**

**Table (14): Chromatographic and spectral data of compound (9)**

| | | |
|---|---|---|
| 1. | $R_f$–values (x100) | 40 ($H_2O$), 58 (6% AcOH), and 32 (BAW). |
| 2. | UV Spectral data $\lambda_{max}$ (nm) MeOH | MeOH: 267, 353.<br>NaOMe: 275, 310, 402.<br>NaOAc: 275, 355.<br>NaOAc / $H_3BO_3$: 271, 355.<br>$AlCl_3$: 272, 408.<br>$AlCl_3$/ HCl: 270, 406 |
| 3. | $^1$H-NMR Spectral data $\delta$ (ppm) (DMSO-$d_6$) room temperature | 6.74 (1H, $s$, H-8), 6.52 (1H, $s$, H-6), 7.89, 7.92 (2H, $d$, $J$= 8 Hz, H-2', H-6'), 6.92, 6.94 (2H, $d$, $J$= 8 Hz,, H-3', H-5'), 4.63 (1H, $d$, $J$= 7.5 Hz, H-1''), 3.18-3.71 ($m$, glucuronic acid protons hidden by water and hydroxyl proton signals) |

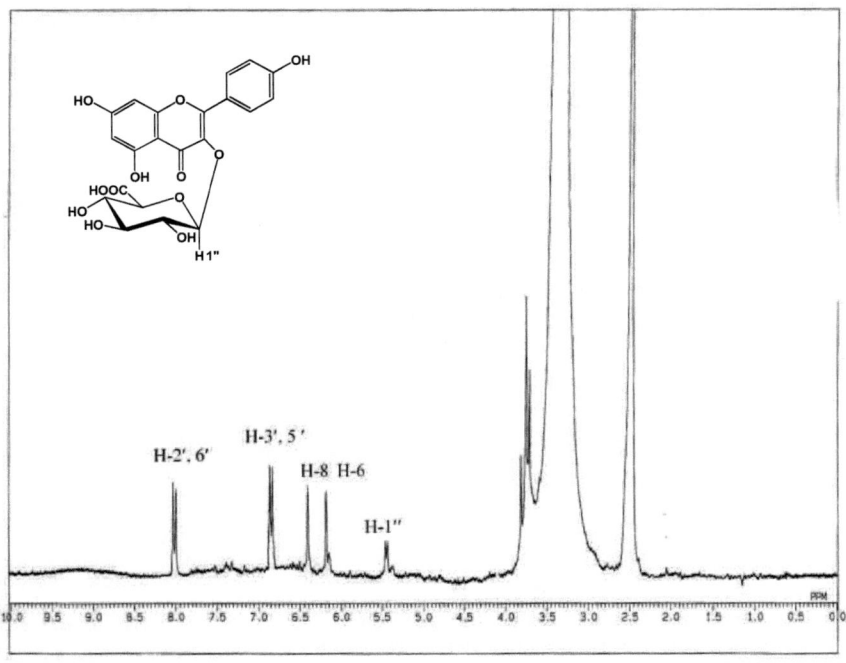

**Fig. (21):** $^1$H-NMR spectrum of compound (9)

## Identification of compound (10): Tamarixetin 3 -$O$-$\beta$ - glucuronide

Chromatographic behaviour (dark brown on PC under UV light), the results of normal, controlled acid and enzymatic hydrolysis (Nawwar *et al.*, 1984e) suggested that **10** (29 mg) is a tamarixetin 3-$O$-glucuronide (CoPC). UV spectral analysis of **10** and its acid hydrolysis product **10a** in methanol and with diagnostic shift reagents (Table 15) indicated that **10a** is the favonol, tamarixetin (positive shifts with all reagents except NaOAc + $H_3BO_3$ and unstable NaOMe spectrum) and that **10** is the 3-glucuronide of **10a** (hypsochromic shift of band I relative to that of **10a** in MeOH and the relatively small $AlCl_3$ shift and unstable NaOMe spectrum). ESI-FTMS (poitive ion) (Fig. 22) of **10**: m/z = 492.4028= $(M+1)^+$ corresponding to a molecular formula of $C_{22}H_{17}O_{12}$. The $^1$H-NMR spectrum of **10** (Fig. 23) and **10a** (Table 15) showed sharp signals overlapping with broad signals from hydroxylic protons. They are in accordance with the proposed structures. The signals of the protons H-6, H-8, H-2', H-5', H-6' of **10** are closely similar to the corresponding signals in the spectrum of **10a**. This is obviously due to the absence of recognizable effect caused by the glucuronide moiety located at position 3. The $^{13}$C-NMR spectra (Fig. 24), (Table 15) confirm the proposed structures for **10** and **10a**. Most of the chemical shift values for **10** are the same as for the tamarixetin aglycone and for β-D-glucupyranouronic acid. The attachment of the sugar moiety to C-3 follows from the upfield shift of the C-3 signal and the downfield shift of the signals of its *ortho* and *para*-related carbons: C-2 and C-9. Similar shifts are well known from the work of (Markham *et al.*, 1978). The β-configuration is derived from the position of the anomeric carbon signal at 100.83 ppm (Markham *et al.*, 1978). In **10** the position of the glucuronide moiety at C-3 is recognized from the upfield shift of the C-3 signal and the large downfield shift of the C-2 signal (all in comparison with **10a**) (Urbatsch *et al.*, 1976). Other resonances in this spectrum exhibited chemical shift values, which were in close agreement to the achieved structure of compound **10** as tamarixetin 3-$O$-β-glucupyranoronide, a natural product, which represents, to the best of our knowledge, a new natural product.

**Compound (10): Tamarixetin 3-*O*-β-glucuronide**

**Table (15): Chromatographic and spectral data of compounds (10 and 10a)**

|   | Compound (10) |
|---|---|
| 1. $R_f$ values (x 100) | 55 ($H_2O$), 37 (HOAc-6), 35 (BAW) |
| 2. UV Spectral Data $\lambda_{max}$ (nm), MeOH | MeOH: 258, 260, 372;<br>NaOMe: 268, 422;<br>NaOAC: 256 (inflection), 274, 312, 360 sh.;<br>NaOAc - $H_3BO_3$: 257, 260 inf., 365;<br>$AlCl_3$: 260, 301inf., 363, 430;<br>$AlCl_3$ + HCl: 259, 300 inf., 360, 424. |
| 3. $^1$H- NMR Spectral Data (DMSO-$d_6$)δ (ppm) | Tamarixetin moiety (Aglycone part):<br>6.19 (1H, *d*, *J* = 2.4 Hz, H-6), 6.38 (1H, *d*, *J* = 2.4 Hz, H-8), 7.30 (d, $J_{meta}$ = 1.7 Hz, H-2'), 6.80 (1H, *d*, *J* = 8.5 Hz, H-5'), 7.39 (1H, *dd*, *J* = 8.5 Hz and 1.7 Hz, H-6'), 3.76 (OMe, s).<br><br>Glucuronic acid moiety (sugar part):<br>5.30 (1H, *d*, *J* = 7 Hz, H-1''), 3.2- 3.4 (*m*, sugar protons) |

| | |
|---|---|
| 4. $^{13}$C-NMR Spectral Data (DMSO-d$_6$)δ (ppm) | Tamarixetin moiety<br>156.32 (C – 2), 132.76 (C – 3), 177.30 (C – 4), 161.09 (C – 5), 98.56 (C – 6), 164.45 (C – 7), 93.74 (C – 8), 156.55 (C – 9), 103.70 (C – 10), 121.76 (C – 1'), 115.02 (C - 2'), 146.81 (C – 3'), 149.21 (C – 4'), 114.07 (C – 5'), 121.15 (C – 6'), 55.69 ( Me-4').<br><br>Glucuronic acid moiety<br>Glucuronic: 100.83(C-1''), 72.18 (C-2''), 74.16 ( C - 3''), 74.41 (C - 4''), 76.17 (C -5''), 171.71 (C - 6''). |
| | Compound (10a), Tamarixetin aglycone |
| 1. $R_f$ values (x 100) | 8 (H$_2$O), 17 (HOAc-6), 83 (BAW) |
| 2. UV Spectral Data λ$_{max}$ (nm), MeOH | MeOH: 255, 268, 369;<br>NaOMe: 268, 422;<br>NaOAC: 253 (inflection), 273, 312, 360 sh.;<br>NaOAc - H$_3$BO$_3$: 255, 265 inf., 368;<br>AlCl$_3$: 268, 301inf., 363, 430;<br>AlCl$_3$ + HCl: 268, 301 inf., 362, 426. |
| 3. $^1$H- NMR Spectral Data (DMSO-d$_6$)δ (ppm) | 6.22 (1H, $d$, $J$= 2 Hz, H-6),<br>6.45 (1H, $d$, $J$=2 Hz, H-8),<br>7.08 (1H, $d$, $J$ =8 Hz, H-5'),<br>7.65 (m, H-2' and H-6'),<br>3.81 ($s$, Me-4'). |
| 4. $^{13}$C-NMR Spectral Data (DMSO-d$_6$)δ (ppm) | 146.2 (C – 2), 136 (C – 3), 175.9 (C – 4), 160.8 (C – 5), 98 (C – 6), 163.9 (C – 7), 93.3 (C – 8), 156.2 (C – 9), 103.0 (C – 10), 123.2 (C – 1'), 114.80 (C - 2'), 146 (C – 3'), 149.01 (C – 4'), 111.50 (C – 5'), 119.40 (C – 6'), 55.8 ( Me-4'). |

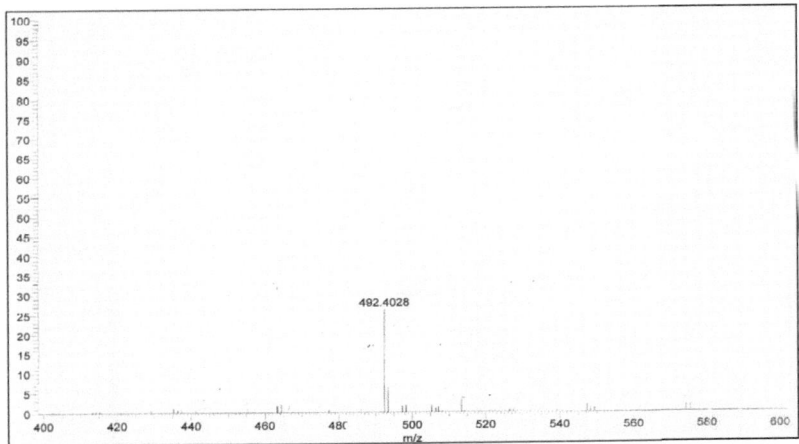

Fig. (22): ESI-MS spectrum of compound (10)

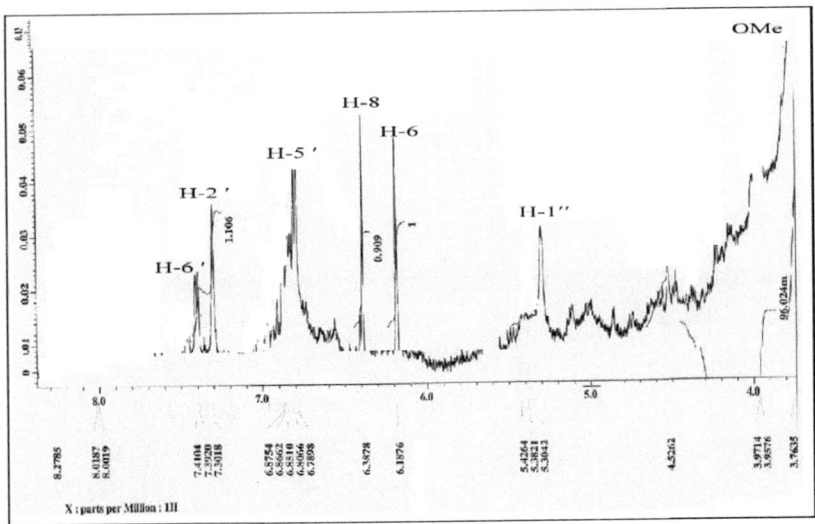

Fig. (23): $^1$H –NMR spectrum of compound (10)

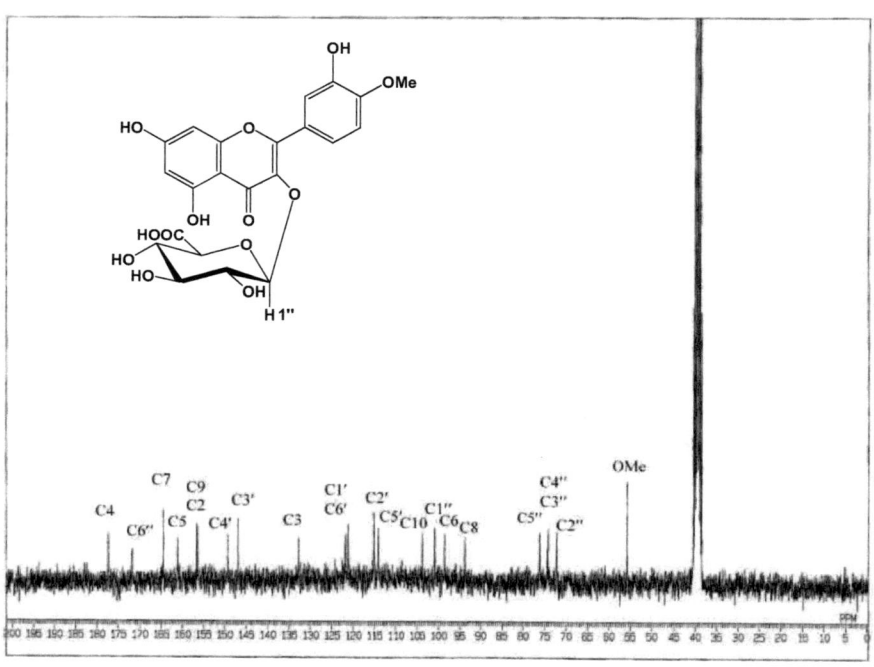

Fig. (24): $^1$H-NMR spectrum of compound (10)

## Fraction VII

Among minor constituents which were shown under UV light on 2DPC of this fraction, two components were found predominant compounds (11) and (12) and appeared as blue coloured spots. 2DPC of this fraction revealed that, both components were found to possess the properties of galloyl esters (pink colour with saturated aqueous $KIO_3$ and intense blue colour with $FeCl_3$ spray reagents).

## Isolation of compounds (11) and (12):

Application of repeated PPC, using $n$-BuOH saturated with water as solvent on the material (1.1 g) of fraction VII (1.89 g, eluted with 50 % MeOH) afforded pure samples of compounds 11 (42 mg) and 12 (49 mg).

## Identification of compound (11), 1, 3-di-*O*-Galloyl-*β*-glucose

Compound 11 (42 mg), isolated as an off-white amorphous powder, was proved through chromatographic; colour reactions (intense blue $FeCl_3$, rosy red colour with $KIO_3$), UV spectral; hydrolytic data, yielding gallic acid and glucose (CoPC) and negative ESI-MS analysis, ([M-H]$^-$ ion at m/z =483, Fig. 11), to be a digalloyl glucose.

Characterization of this constituent was completed by $^1H$ and $^{13}C$ analysis as well as by comparing the received data with those reported for similar galloyl glucoses (Haddock et al., 1982a). The $^1$H-NMR spectrum of 11, (Fig. 26) revealed two aromatic proton singlets (Table 16), at δ 6.98 and 6.97 ppm assignable to the two existing galloyl moieties. The spectrum also showed in the sugar region, two clearly resolved downfield proton resonances, the most down field of which was found to resonate at δ 5.6 ppm ($d$, $J$=8 Hz), attributable to a β-configurated anomeric glucose proton. The second downfield sugar proton resonance was recognized at δ 5.0 3 ppm ($t$, $J$= 8Hz). The significant downfield shifts, recognized for these two sugar resonance (in comparison with the resonances of the corresponding protons in free β-glucose) indicated that the hydroxyl groups, geminal to these protons are galloylated, thus proving the structure to be 1,3-di-*O*-galloyl-β-glucose.

$^{13}$C-NMR spectrum of 11, (Fig. 27) exhibited carbon resonances (Table 16) which were in accordance with this structure. The β-anomeric carbon was recognized from the resonance at δ 94.1 ppm. The most downfield sugar resonance located at δ 78.2 ppm is obviously due to the galloylated sugar carbon, C-3. Galloylation at C-3 also followed from the upfield shifts of the resonances of C-2 and C-4, compared to the resonances of the corresponding carbons in the spectrum of free β-glucose. These β-effects have been previously observed in similar cases. The presence of two galloyl moieties in **11** follows from the two carboxylic carbonyl carbon resonances, recorded in this spectrum at δ 165.4 and 166.2 ppm. Other chemical shifts of the resonances of the remaining galloyl and glucose carbons in this spectrum were in agreement with the achieved structure of **11** as 1, 3-di-*O*-galloyl-β-glucose (Jiang *et al.*, 2001)

**Compound (11): 1, 3-di-*O*-Galloyl-β-glucose**

**Table (16): Chromatographic and spectral data of compound (11)**

| | |
|---|---|
| 1. $R_f$ values (x 100) | 65 ($H_2O$), 73 (HOAc), 38 (BAW) |
| 2. UV spectral data $\lambda_{max}$ (nm) | 278 |
| 3. $^1$H- NMR spectral data (DMSO-$d_6$) $\delta$ (ppm) | Glucose moiety<br>5.6 (1H, d, J= 8 Hz, H-1)<br>5.03 (1H, t, J=8 Hz, H-3)<br>3.1-4.0 (m, H-2,4,5,6)<br>Galloyl moiety<br>6.97(2H, s, H-2' and H-6'), 6.99(2H, s, H-2" and H-6") |
| 4. $^{13}$C-NMR spectral data (DMSO-$d_6$) $\delta$ (ppm) | Glucose<br>94.1 (C-1), 77.1(C-2), 78.2(C-3), 70.5(C-4), 71.6(C-5), 61.1(C-6)<br><br>Galloyl moieties<br>120.3,119(C-1',1"),110.1,110,109,108 (C-2',6',2",6"),145.8,145.7(C3',5',3",5"), 138.7,139.6(C-4' 4"),165.4,166.2(C=O) |

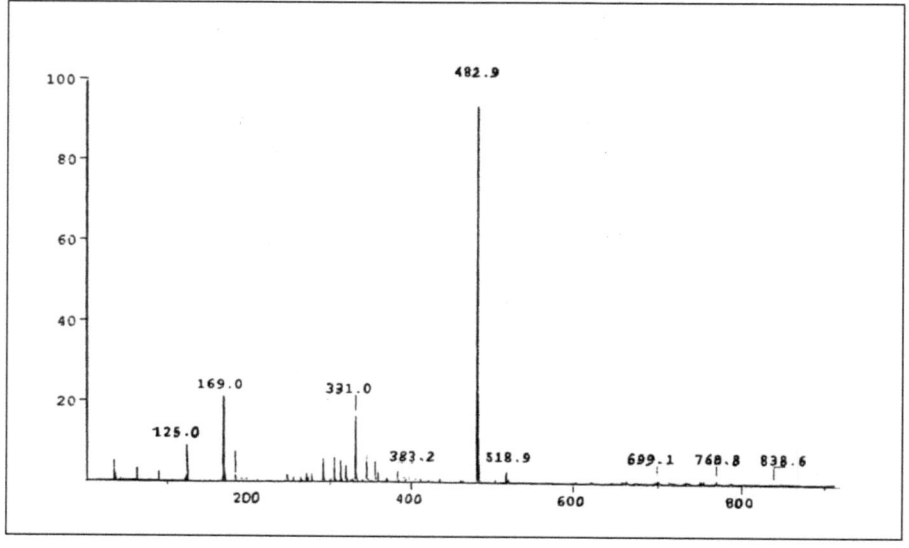

**Fig. (25): ESI-MS spectrum of compound (11)**

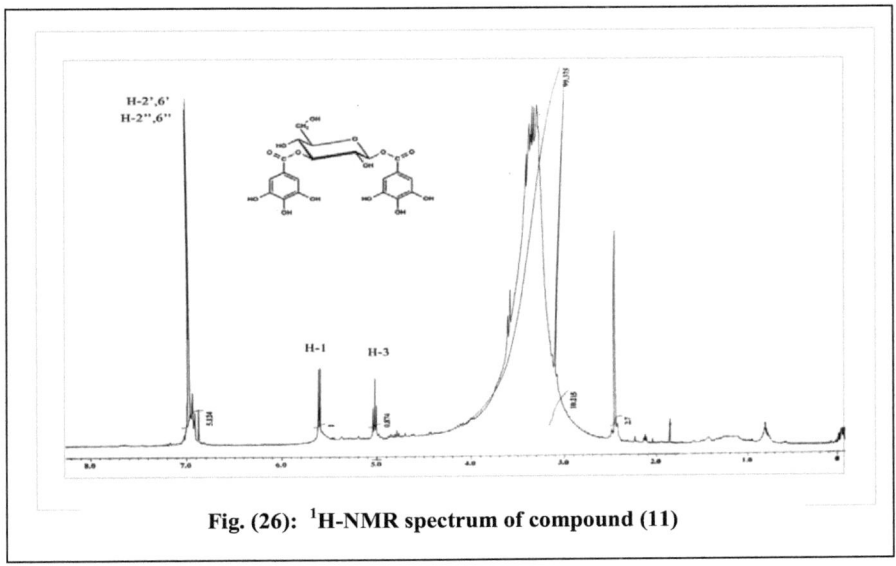

**Fig. (26):** $^1$H-NMR spectrum of compound (11)

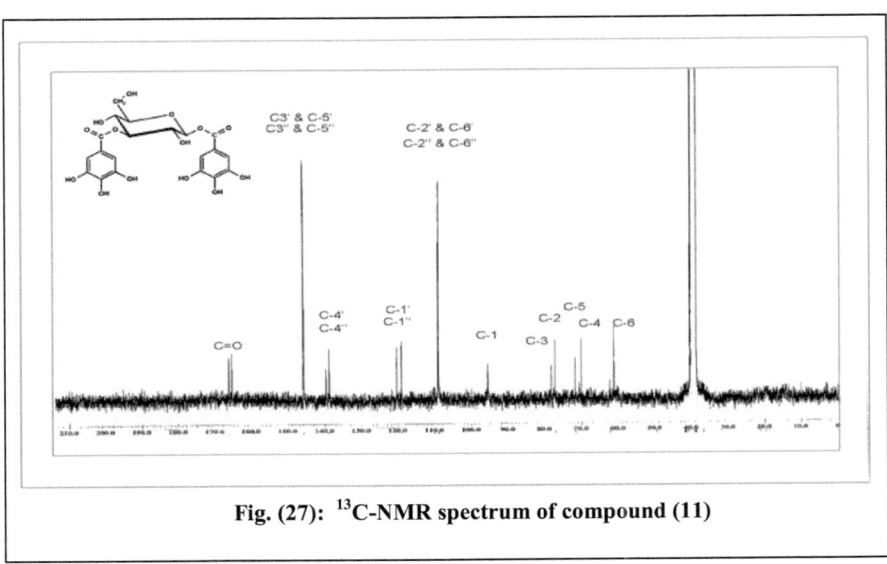

**Fig. (27):** $^{13}$C-NMR spectrum of compound (11)

## Identification of compound (12): 2, 4-di-*O*-Galloyl (α/β) glucopyranose

Compound **12** (49 mg) was obtained as an amorphous powder which possesses galloyl ester-like characters [intense blue color with $FeCl_3$, rosy red color with $KIO_3$ (Haddock *et al.*, 1982a) and UV spectral maximum in MeOH at 274 nm]. ESIMS analysis (Negative mode) established that compound **12** was a digalloyl glucose with a Mr of 484 (m/z = 483, [M H]⁻ as was confirmed by HRESIMS, m/z: 483.3563 (calc.: 483.3572) for molecular formula $C_{20}H_{20}O_{14}$. On normal acid hydrolysis (2N aqueous HCl at 100 C for 3 hours) **12** yielded gallic acid (CoPC, UV, $^1H$ and, $^{13}C$-NMR spectral analyses) together with glucose (CoPC), while on controlled acid hydrolysis (0.5 N aq. HCl, 100oC, 3 hours) it gave, beside glucose and gallic acid (CoPC), an intermediate **12a** which was extracted from the hydolysate by EtOAc and purified by preparative paper chromatography. This was shown to have a Mr of 332 (negative ESIMS: [M - H]⁻, m/z 331) and UV spectral maximum in MeOH at 273 nm, thus suggesting its structure to be a monogalloyl glucose. To determine the site of attachment of the two-galloyl moieties to the glucose core in the molecule of **12**, $^1H$-NMR spectral analysis was then carried out. The spectrum, recorded in DMSO-$d_6$ revealed, characteristic singlets of the galloyl moieties at 6.93, 6.94, 6.95 and 6.97 two different patterns of proton signals belonging to an α/β anomeric mixture of disubstituted glucose, whereby a pair of doublets, centered at δ 5.19 ($J = 3.5$ Hz) and at 4.70 ($J = 8$ Hz) were recognized and assigned to the α- and β-anomeric glucose protons, respectively, thus indicating a free anomeric OH group. The spectrum also showed two downfield glucose proton resonances at 4.62 (*dd*, $J = 3.5$ Hz and J = 8 Hz) and at 4.72 (*t*, $J = 8$ Hz) assignable to the H-2 glucose protons in both α- and β-anomers, respectively. The downfield location of both resonances is clearly, due to galloylation of their geminal OH groups. This assignment was based on the observation that the double doublet mode of splitting of the signal located at 4.62 is typical of an axial H-2 proton in α-$^4C_1$-glucose core, being coupled to both the α-anomeric equatorial proton ($J = 3.5$ Hz) and to the axial H-3 proton ($J = 8$ Hz) of the same moiety. Galloylation at 4-position of the glucose core was evidenced by the two low field proton signals located at δ 4.83 (*t*, $J = 8$ Hz) and 4.72 (*t*, $J = 8$ Hz), assignable to H-4α and H-4β, respectively, an assignment which was confirmed by measurement of a $^1H$-$^1H$-COSY spectrum. In addition, the values of the above coupling constants indicated that the α- and β-glucose cores of **12** are adopting a $^4C_1$ conformer. The weight of evidence given above, proved that compound **12** is 2, 4-di-O-galloyl-(α/β)-$^4C_1$-glucose. Final proof of structure was then achieved through $^{13}C$-NMR spectral analysis which afforded a spectrum containing essentially double signals for most of the glucose and galloyl carbons. Resonances were assigned by comparison with the $^{13}$C NMR data, reported for similar galloyl glucoses (Nawwar and Hussein, 1994; Nawwar et al., 1984a) as well as by consideration of the known α- and β-effect caused by esterifying the sugar hydroxl groups (Nawwar and Hussein, 1994). In the received spectrum, the α- and β-anomeric carbon signals were readily identified from their characteristic chemical shift values (δ ppm 89.7, C-1α and 94.8, C-1β). Attachment of one of the galloyl moiety to C-2 of the glucose core followed from the β-upfield shift recognized for the resonances of both the vicinal C-1 and C-3 carbons (β-effect) and from the downfield shift of the resonances of the C-2 carbon (α-effect). Attachment of the second galloyl moiety to C-4 of glucose was evidenced by the β-upfield shift recognized for the vicinal carbon (C-3 and C-5) resonances [all in comparison with the chemical shifts of the corresponding carbon resonances in the spectrum of unsubstituted α/β glucopyranos]. In both anomers, the resonances of C-2 was found to be shifted downfield (α-effect) at δ 75.8 (C-2-α) and 76.7 (C-2-β), while those of C-4 were shifted downfield to 71.6 (C-4-α) and 73.8 (C-4-β). Other resonances in this spectrum exhibited chemical shift values which were in accordance with the proposed structure. All assignments were confirmed by HSQC and HMBC experiments. Furthermore, the measured chemical shift values of the glucose carbon resonances proved that this moiety existed in the pyranose form, thus confirming the final structure of **12** to be 2, 4-di-*O*-galloyl-(α/β)-$^4$C$_1$-glucopyranose, a secondary metabolite which has not reported before in literature.

**Compound 12: 2, 4-di-*O*-Galloyl - $^4$C$_1$-(α/β)- glucopyranose**

## Table (17): Chromatographic and spectral data of compounds 12 and 12a

| | Compound 12 |
|---|---|
| 1. $R_f$ values (x 100) | 55 ( $H_2O$), 63 (HOAc), 42 (BAW) |
| 2. UV spectral data λmax (nm) | 274 |
| 3. $^1$H- NMR spectral data (DMSO-d6)δ (ppm) | α-Glucose moiety<br>19 (*d, J*=3.5 Hz, H-l),<br>4.62 (*dd, J*=8 and 3.5 Hz, H-2). 3.99 (*t, J*=8 Hz, H-3). 4.83(*t, J*=8 Hz, H-4), 3.90 (m, H-5), 3.3-3.6 (m, H2-6 proton overlapped with water signal)<br><br>β-glucose moiety<br>4.70 (*d, J*=8 Hz, H-1), 4.72 (*t, J*=8 Hz, H-2), 4.72 (*t,J*=8 Hz, H-4), 3.76 (m, H-5), 3.3-3.6 (m, overlapped with water signal, H2-6)<br><br>α-Glucose moiety<br>89.7 (C-l), 75.8 (C-2), 72.4 (C-3), 71.4 (C-4)', 70.3 (C-5), 61.0 (C-6);<br><br>β-glucose moiety<br>94.7 (C-l), 76.7 (C-2), 75.5 (C-3). 71.8 (C-4), 74.9 (C-5). 61.1 (C- 6); |
| 4. $^{13}$C-NMR spectral data (DMSO-d6)δ (ppm) | Galloyl moieties<br>120.5, 119.9, 119.8 (C-l), 109.6, 109.4(C-2and C-6). 146, 1, 146.0, 145.9 (C-3 and C-5). 139, 1, 139.0, 138.8, 138.0 (C-4), 166.2, 165.9, 165.6, 165.1 (C = O). |
| | Compound 12a |
| 1. $R_f$ values (x 100) | 71 ($H_2O$),74 (HOAc) , 64( BAW) |
| 2. UV spectral data λmax (nm) | 273 |

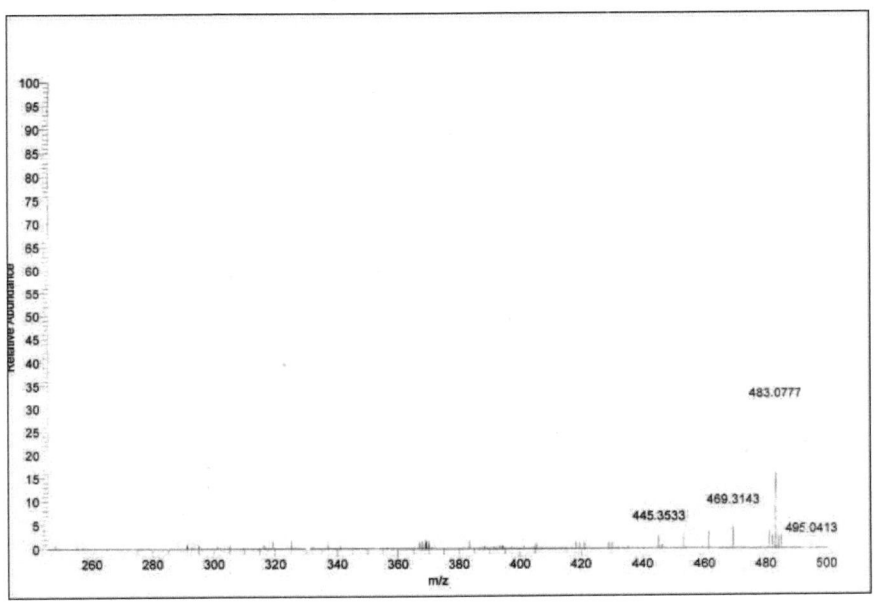

Fig. (28): ESI/MS spectrum of compound (12)

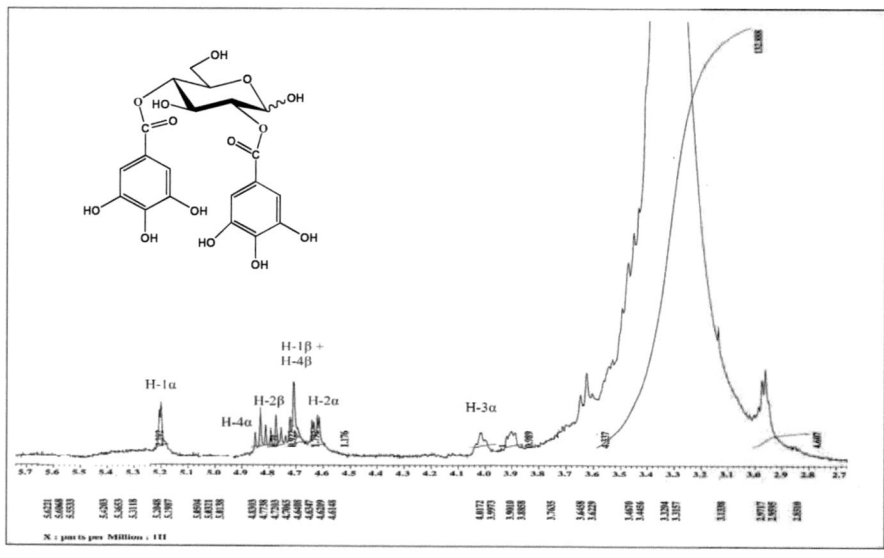

Fig. (29): $^1$H-NMR spectrum of sugar protons of compound (12)

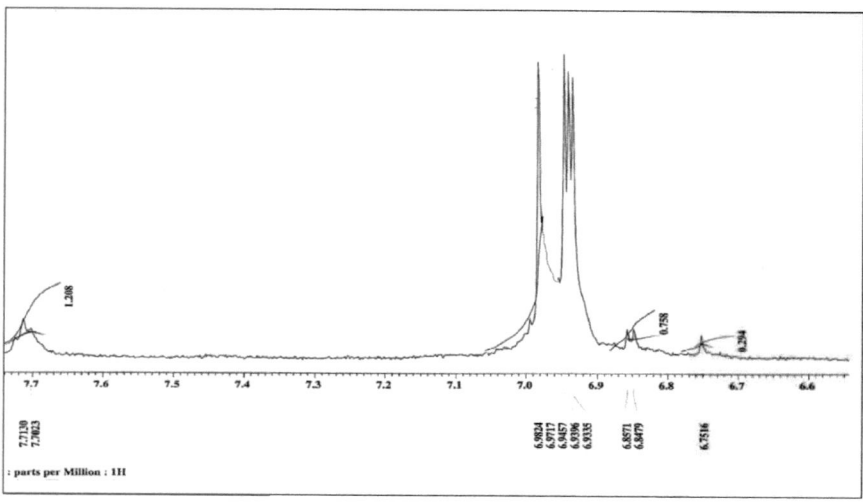

Fig. (30): $^1$H-NMR spectrum of aromatic protons of compound (12)

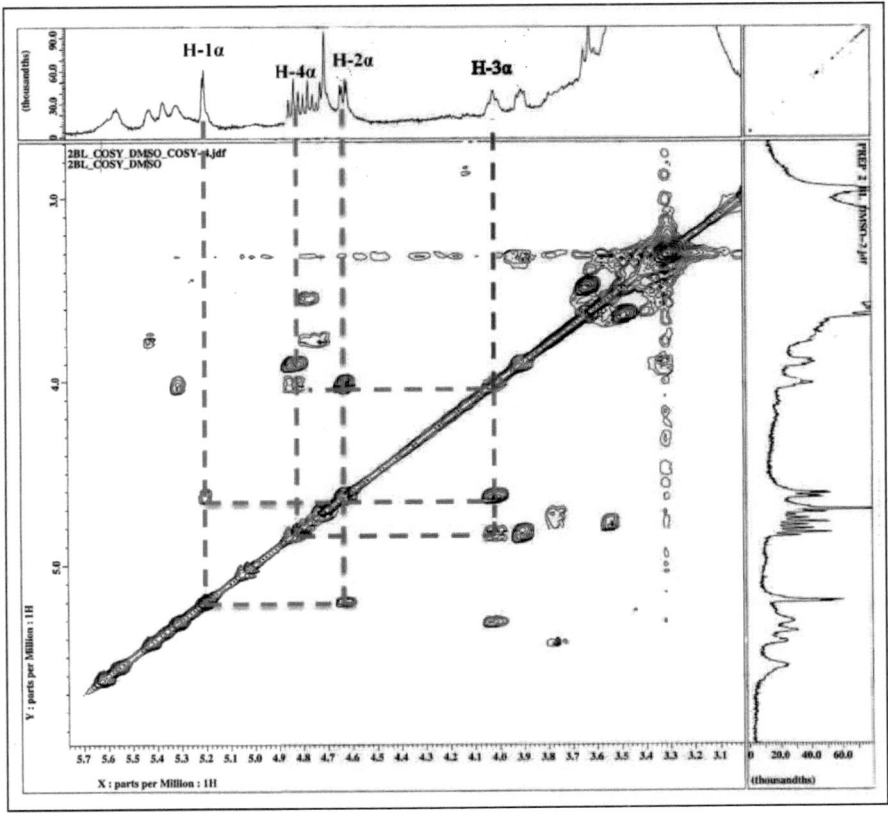

**Fig. (31):** $^1$H-$^1$H COSY spectrum of compound (12)

## Fraction VIII

The light brown amorphous material of this fraction was found to contain one major phenolic component belonging to gallotannins (deep blue color on PC under UV light, intense blue color with $FeCl_3$ and rosy red with $KIO_3$).

## Isolation of compound (13)

Compound **13** was obtained pure (52 mg) by repeated precipitation (thrice) from a concentrated acetone solution of 302 mg of fraction VIII (1.58 g, eluted with 60 % MeOH) by ether.

## Identification of compound (13): 2, 6-di-O-Galloyl-($\alpha/\beta$)-$^4C_1$- glucopyranose

Pure material of **13**, a non-crystalline amorphous white powder (52 mg) appeared on PC as a dark blue spot, which gave an intense blue color with $FeCl_3$ and a rosy red color with $KIO_3$. Compound **13** possessed a UV absorption maximum in MeOH at 275 nm (Table 6), a $Mr$ of 484 mu (negative ESI-MS: $[M-H]^-$ : 483), (Fig. 32) and gave on complete acid hydrolysis gallic acid and glucose ( CoPC).

On partial hydrolysis **13** gave, beside glucose and gallic acid (CoPC), an intermediate **13a**, which was separated pure through Prep. PC, using BAW as solvent. **13a** was shown to have a $Mr$ of 332 mu (negative FAB-MS: $[M-H]^-$ : 331) (Fig. 33) and $\lambda_{max}$ (in MeOH) at 273 nm (Table 18), thus suggesting its structure to be a mono galloyl glucose. The site of attachment between the galloyl moiety and the glucose core in the molecule of **13a** was determined by $^1$H-NMR analysis (Fig. 35) (Nawwar and Hussein, 1994) , to be at the glucose carbon no. 6.

The above given data suggested that the parent compound **13** should be a digalloyl glucose in which one of the galloyl moieties is located at carbon No.6 of the glucose moiety. To determine the site of attachment of the second galloyl moiety, $^1$H-NMR spectral analysis of **13**, (DMSO-d6, room temperature), was undertaken. The received spectrum (Fig. 34) (Table 18) showed, two different patterns of proton signals belonging to an $\alpha/\beta$ anomeric mixture of digalloyl glucose, whereby a pair of doublets, centered at $\delta$ 5.14 ($J$ = 3.5 Hz) and 4.66 ( $J$ = 8 Hz) were recognized and assigned to the $\alpha$- and $\beta$-anomeric glucose protons respectively. The spectrum also, showed two downfield glucose proton signals, at $\delta$4.59 (dd, $J$= 3.5 Hz and $J$= 8  Hz) and $\delta$ 4.65 (t, $J$= 8 Hz), assignable to H-2 protons of both $\alpha$- and $\beta$-anomers, respectively. This assignment was based on the fact that the double doublet mode of splitting of the signal located at δ 4.59 ppm is typical for an axial H-2 proton, in an α- anomeric equatorial proton ($J= 3.5$ Hz) and to the axial H-3 proton ($J= 8$ Hz) of the same moiety. On the other hand, galloylation at No. 6 of both glucose anomers of compound **13** was further evidenced by the low-field pair of doublets at δ 4.43 and 4.41 ppm ($J= 12.5$ Hz) as well as by the low-field pair of double doublets at δ 4.31 and 4.32 ppm (both with $J=12.5$ Hz and $J=4.5$ Hz), assignable to methylinic H-6a and H-6b protons in both anomers (all in comparison with the protons chemical shifts, reported for D-(α/β)-glucopyranose ( De Bruyn et al., 1977). In addition, the measured coupling constants indicate that the glucose core of **13** is adopting a $^4C_1$ conformation (De Bruyn et al., 1977).

The above given data confirmed that compound **13** is derived through the galloylation of the glucose hydroxyls located at position No.2 and 6 to yield 2,6-di-*O*-galloyl-(α/β)-$^4C_1$-glucose. The final structure of compound **13** has been achieved through $^{13}$C-NMR spectral analysis which affored a spectrum (Fig. 36) containing almost a double signal for most of the sugar and galloyl protons. Resonance recorded in this spectrum were assigned by comparison with spectra of similar galloylated glucoses and those of α- and β- glucose itself (Nawwar et al., 1984c), as well as by consideration of the known α- and β-effect (Nawwar et al., 1984d) caused by the galloylation of a sugar hydroxyl group. The α- and β-anomeric carbon signals were readily identified by their characteristic chemical shift values (δ 89.6, C-α and 94.9, C-β), while the two overlapped most upfield resonance were assigned to the galloylated glucose carbons No. 6 (δ 63.6, C-6, in both anomers).

The attachment of the second galloyl moiety to position No. 2 of the sugar followed from the β-up-field effect recognized for the resonances of the vicinal C-1, as well as C-3 carbon [all in comparison with the corresponding resonances in the spectrum of (α/β)-glucose itself ( De Bruyn et al., 1977). Carbons No.2, themselves were found resonating down-field at δ 75.2 ppm ($C_2$-α) and 76.5 ppm ($C_2$-β) due to the α- effect of the galloyl moiety. Other resonance in this spectrum exhibited chemical shift values, which were in accordance with the achieved structure of compound **13**. Consequently, compound **13** is 2,6-di-*O*-galloyl-(α/β)-$^4C_1$- glucopyranose (Nawwar and Hussein, 1994).

**Compound 13: 2, 6-di-$O$-Galloyl-($\alpha/\beta$)-$^4C_1$- glucopyranose**

**Table (18): Chromatographic and spectral data of compound 13 and 13a**

| | | |
|---|---|---|
| 1. | $R_f$ values (x 100) | 60 ($H_2O$), 68 (HOAc-6), 44 (BAW) |
| 2. | UV Spectral Data<br>$\lambda_{max}$ (nm), MeOH | 275 |
| 3. | $^1$H- NMR Spectral Data<br>(DMSO-$d_6$)$\delta$ (ppm) | $\alpha$-Glucose:<br>5.14 *(d, J =3.5 Hz, H-1)*,<br>4.59 *(dd, J =8 and 3.5 Hz, H-2)*,<br>3.80 *(t, J =8 Hz, H-3)*,<br>3.46-3.59 *(m, H-4)*, 3.95 *(m, H-5)*,<br>4.43 *(d, J = 12.5 Hz, H-6)*, 4.31 *(dd, J = 12.5 Hz and 4.5 Hz, H-6')*.<br><br>$\beta$-Glucose:<br>4.66 *(d, J =8 Hz. H-1)*,<br>4.65 *(t, J =8 Hz, H-2)*,<br>3.78(t, J =8 Hz, H-3), 3.46-3.59 *(m, H-4)*, 3.95 *(m, H-5)*. 4.41 *(d, J = 12.5 Hz, H-6)*, 4.32 *(dd. J= 12.5 and 4.5 Hz, H-6')*. |
| 4. | $^{13}$C-NMR Spectral Data<br>(DMSO-$d_6$)$\delta$ (ppm) | Galloyl moieties in $\alpha$- & $\beta$-anomers:<br>6.97 (s), 6.98 (s), 6.99 (s), 7.01 (s). |

|  | α-Glucose:<br>89.6 (C-l), 75.2 (C-2), 70.6 (C-3), 69.4 (C-4), 69.4 (C-5), 63.6 (C-6).<br><br>β-Glucose:<br>94.9 (C-l), 76.5 (C-2), 75.5 (C-3), 70.3 (C-4), 70.9 (C-5). 63.6 (C-6).<br><br>Galloyl moieties in α- & β-anomers:<br>117.62, 117.63 (C-l), 108.75, 109.1 (C-2 and C-6), 146.24, 146.35 (C-3 and C-5), 141.7, 141.8 (C-4), 165.5, 166.3, 166.34 (C=O). |
|---|---|

|  | Compound 13a |
|---|---|
| 1. $R_f$ values (x 100) | 67 ($H_2O$), 75 (HOAc-6), 33 (BAW) |
| 2. UV Spectral Data<br>$\lambda_{max}$ (nm), MeOH | 273 |
| 3. $^1$H- NMR Spectral Data (DMSO-$d_6$) δ (ppm) | α-Glucose: 5.10 *(d, J=3.5* Hz, H-l), 3.50-3.90 *(m,* H-2, H-3 and H-4), 3.92 *(m,* H-5), 4.38 *(d, J=* 12.5 Hz, H-6), 4.25 *(dd, J=* 12.5 and 4.5 Hz, H-6').<br><br>β-Glucose: 4.60 *(d, J* = 8 Hz, H-l), 3.50-3.90 *(m,* H-2, H-3 and H-4), 3.93 *(m,* H-5), 4.42 *(d, J=* 12.5 Hz, H-6), 4.30 (dd, *J=* 12.5 and 4.5 Hz, H-6').<br><br>Galloyl moieties in α- & β-anomers: 6.99 (s) and 7.00 (s). |

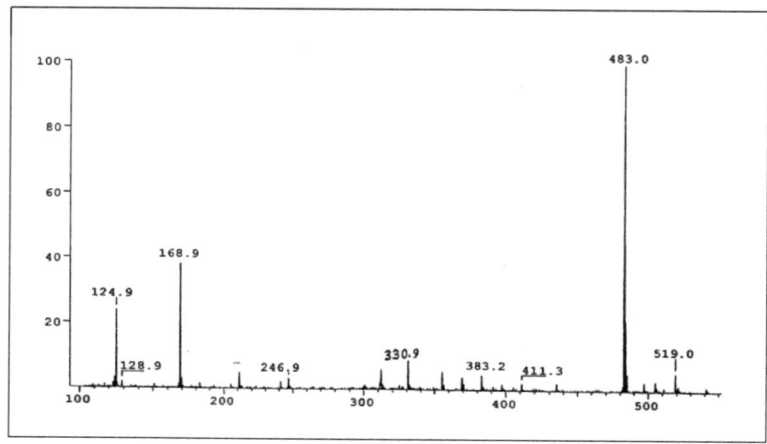

Fig. (32): Negative ESI/MS spectrum of compound (13)

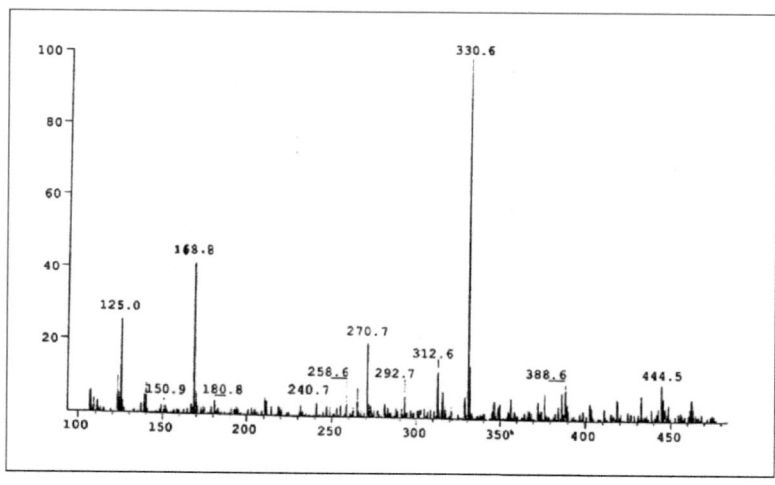

Fig. (33): Negative FAB – MS of compound (13a)

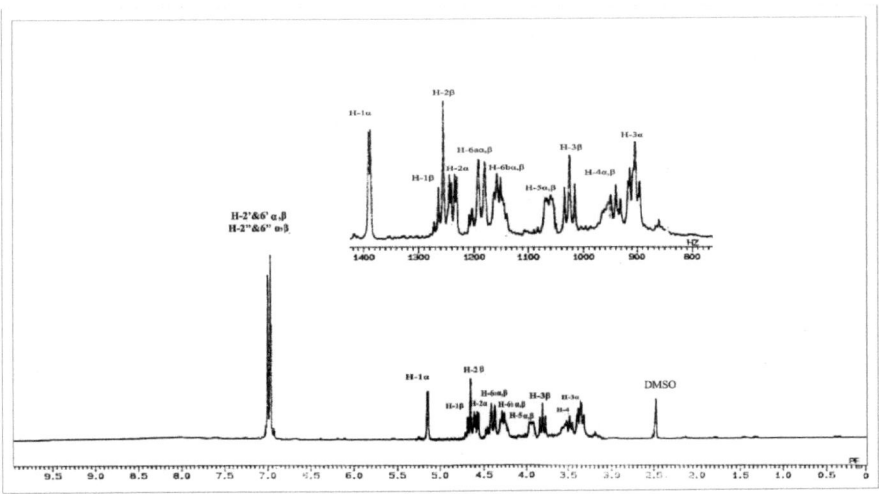

Fig. (34): $^1$H-NMR spectrum of compound (13)

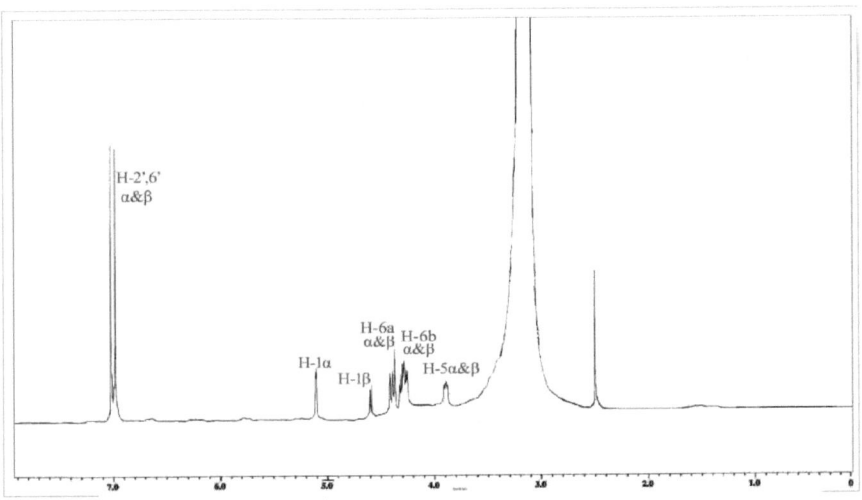

Fig. (35): $^1$H-NMR spectrum of compound (13a)

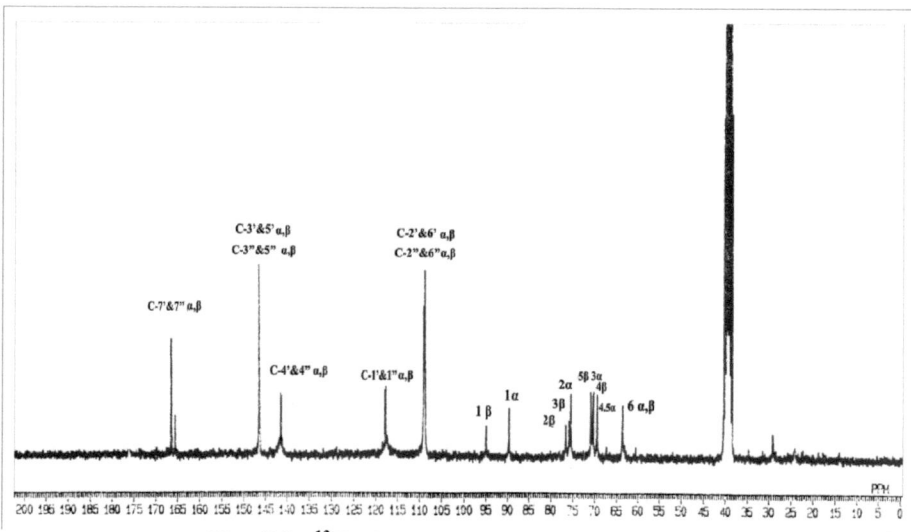

**Fig. (36):** $^{13}C$ – NMR spectrum of compound (13)

## Fraction IX

Fraction IV showed by 2DPC major component (**14**). Compound (**14**) appears as dark blue spot under short UV light on PC, which turned intense blue in day light on spraying with $FeCl_3$ spray reagent. Also, it gives rose violet color when sprayed with nitrous acid spray reagent, thus suggesting the ellagitannin character (Gupta et al., 1982).

## Isolation of compound (14)

Extraction of 406 mg material of fraction IX (2.5 g, eluted with 70 % MeOH) with EtOAc, while hot, followed by filtration, concentration of the filtrate, cooling to room temp. and addition of ether led to precipitation of compound **14** which was filtered off and re-precipitated (thrice) to give a pure sample (90 mg).

## Identification of compound (14): Tamarixellagic acid

Compound **14**, isolated as a light brown amorphous powder (90 mg) was found to possess chromatographic properties, colour reactions (dark blue with $FeCl_3$ and violet with nitrous acid spray reagents on PC) and UV spectral data consistent with an ellagitannin (Table 16). It exhibited a molecular ion peak at $[M+H]^+$ 955 in positive ESI-MS (Fig. 38) and at $[M-H]^+$ 953 in negative ESI-MS, corresponding to a $M_r$ of 954.

On complete acid hydrolysis (30 mg was refluxed with 25 ml, 2 N aq. HCl, 100°C, 3 hr), **14** yielded glucose ( gallic, ellagic and dehydrodigallic acids (Co-PC). The released ellagic acid, precipitated from the cold aqueous hydrolysate was fully characterized through UV, $^1H$ and $^{13}C$-NMR spectral analysis (Nawwar et al., 1994b), while the released gallic and dehydrodigallic acids were individually separated by polyamide column of their ethyl acetate extract, using $H_2O$-EtOH mixtures of decreasing polarities (20 and 40%, respectively) for elution. UV, $^1H$ and $^{13}C$-NMR spectral analysis confirmed the identity of the received data.

On controlled acid hydrolysis (35 mg was refluxed together with 25 ml of 0.1 N aq. HCl, 100°C, 3 hr), **14** yielded, among other products, 4,6-O-hexahydroxybiphenoylglucose (co-PC, UV spectral data and positive ESI-MS: 483 [M+H]+; Mr 482 (Fig.37); together with an ellagitannin intermediate **14a** which appeared on 2DPC as a dark blue spot on PC in UV light turning dark blue when sprayed with FeCl3, and violet on spraying with nitrous acid (Gupta et al., 1982). A pure amorphous sample of **14a**, obtained through preparative PC of the ethyl acetate extract of the controlled acid hydrolysis products, was found to possess UV spectral data similar to that of **14**.

Positive and negative ESI-MS of **14a** showed the molecular ion peaks, $[M+H]^+$ 803 (Fig. 39) and $[M-H]^-$ 801(Fig.40), respectively, thus proving a $M_r$ of 802. Hence, **14a** is formed through the mono-esterification of 4, 6-O-hexahydroxybiphenoylglucose moiety with a dehydrodigallic acid moiety. This assumption was then proved through complete acid hydrolysis of **14a** to yield glucose, ellagic and dehydrodigallic acids (co-PC). Consequently, **14a** is 3-O-mono-dehydrodigallicmonocarboxyloyl 4, 6-(S) hexahydroxydiphenoyl-$(\alpha/\beta)$-$^4C_1$,-glucopyranose and **14** is the monogalloyl derivative of **14a**.

To find out the site of attachment of the galloyl and dehydrodigalloyl moiety to the 4,6-hexahydroxybiphenoylglucose moiety to form **14**. $^1$H-NMR spectral analysis was then engaged (Fig.41) (Table 19). The spectrum revealed two distinct patterns of proton signals belonging to substituted α- and β-glucose anomers. Each pattern was found to contain well separated signals of the seven-spin system belonging to a distinct glucose anomer. The spectrum also showed one pair of singlets in the aromatic region for the galloyl moieties (one for each anomer), as well as two pairs of singlets for the hexahydroxybiphenoyl protons (one pair for one moiety in each anomer). The characteristic pattern of dehydrodigallic acid proton signals has revealed itself twice in this spectrum. The appearance of two signals for each distinct proton in **14** proved the presence of a free anomeric glucose hydroxyl group, which restricts the site of attachments of the galloyl and dehydrodigalloyl moieties to the glucose positions 2 and 3.

The ambiguity in determining the site of attachments between the galloyl, dehydrodigalloyl and the 4,6-hexahydroxybiphenoyl glucose moieties to form **14** was then unravelled through measurement of $^1$H-NMR spectrum of the intermediate **14a** (Fig.42) (Table 19) and the subsequent comparison between the spectrum and that of **14**. This comparison has shown the disappearance of the galloyl proton signals from the spectrum of **14a** which was accompanied by a large upfield shift of the H-2-α and H-2-β glucose proton resonances on comparison with the positions of both signals in the spectrum of **14** (Table 19). The recognition that the remaining sugar and phenolic proton signals in the spectrum of **14a** have almost the same chemical shift values and multiplicities as those of the corresponding signals in **14**, confirmed that the galloyl moiety which was released from the parent compound during controlled acid hydrolysis to produce the intermediate **14a** was esterifying the glucose at C-2, leaving the OH at C-3 to be esterified by one of the carboxylic groups of the dehydrodigalloyl moiety, as was concluded from the downfield positions of the geminal H-3- α and H-3-β-glucose proton signals in the spectra of both **14** and **10a** (incomparison with the corresponding signals in the spectrum of α- and β-glucose (De Bruyn et al., 1977). Thus, **14** is a (S)-4, 6-hexahydroxybiphenoyl-(α / β)-glucose which is esterified at positions 2 and 3 of its glucose core by galloyl and dehydrodigalloyl moieties, respectively.

The $^{13}$C-NMR analysis (Fig.43) (Table 19) of **14** has confirmed this structure. As expected, the spectrum exhibited double signals for each carbon. The α- and β-anomers were recognized from the downfield anomeric glucose carbon resonances at δ 89.5 and 95.3 ppm, respectively, while the most upfield signal at δ 62.5 was assigned to the C-6 glucose carbon in both anomers. Assignments of the remaining glucose carbon signals were aided by comparison with the recorded chemical shifts of 2,3-di-O-galloyl-( α / β)-$^4C_1$-glucopyranose (Nawwar et al., 1984a), as well as with those reported for galloylated 4,6-O-hexahydroxybiphenoylglucoses (De Bruyn et al., 1977; Nonaka et al., 1984). Presence of only one galloyl moiety in **14** followed from the two galloyl C=O carbon resonances (one for each anomer) at δ 165.4 and 165.3 ppm, while the presence of a dehydrodigalloyl moiety was apparent from the appearance of the typical dehydrodigallic acid pattern of carbon signals (twice). However, one of the carboxyl carbons of the latter moiety has revealed its signal twice at δ 162.6 and 162.4 ppm, a location, which is upfield when compared with that of the free dehydrodigallic acid carboxyl carbon signals. This shift is obviously due to the esterification of this carboxyl group with the alcoholic glucose OH group at position 3. Furthermore, the measured chemical shift values of the sugar carbon signals confirmed that the sugar core exists in the pyranose form. Precise determination of the final structure of the molecule was achieved through the comparison of the $^1$H- and $^{13}$C-NMR of **14**, (Fig. 72 and 74) with those of tamarixellagic acid (Nawwar et al., 1994a). Consequently, **14** is 2-O-galloyl-3-$O$-(3, 4, 5, 6, 7 pentahydroxybiphenyl ether-$8_a$-carboxylic acid-1-carboxyloyl)-(S)-4,6-hexahydroxybiphenoyl-($\alpha / \beta$)-$^4C_1$-glucopyranose.

β-form

**Compound (14): 2-$O$-Galloyl-3-$O$-(3, 4, 5, 6,7 pentahydroxybiphenyl ether-$8_a$-carboxylic acid-1-carboxyloyl)-(S)-4,6-hexahydroxybiphenoyl-( $\alpha / \beta$)-$^4C_1$-glucopyranose (Tamarixellagic acid)**

**Table (19): Chromatographic and spectral data of compound (14) and its hydrolysate**

| | Compound (14) |
|---|---|
| 1. $R_f$ values (x 100) | 40($H_2O$), 53 (HOAc-6), 47 (BAW)<br>4,6-HHDP-glucose:<br>55($H_2O$), 65 (HOAc-6), 22 (BAW)<br>Compound (14a):<br>47($H_2O$), 61 (HOAc-6), 36 (BAW) |
| 2. UV Spectral Data $\lambda_{max}$ (nm), MeOH | Compound (14):<br>273<br>4,6-HHDP-glucose:<br>267<br>Compound (14a):<br>273 |
| 3. $^1$H- NMR Spectral Data (DMSO-$d_6$)δ (ppm) | Compound (14):<br>α-glucose moiety:<br>5.28 (d, J = 2.5 Hz, H–1–α), 4.88 (m, H–2–α), 5.68 (t, J = 8 Hz, H–3–α), 4.88 (m, H – 4 – α), 4.5 (m, H–5–α), 5.16 (m, H–6–α), 3.78 (d, J = 12 Hz, H–6'–α).<br><br>β-glucose moiety:<br>4.84 (d, J = 8 Hz, H –1– β ), 4.98 (m, H – 2 – β), 5.42 (t, J = 8 Hz, H –3–β), 4.88 (m, H–4–β), 4.15 (m, H–5–β ), 5.16 (m, H–6–β), 3.72 (d, J = 12 Hz, H–6'–β).<br><br>galloyl moieties in α- and β- anomers:<br>6.75, 6.83(each s, H–2 and H–6 in both moieties). |

Aromatic dehydrodigallicmonocarboxyloyl moiety in α- and β- anomers:
6.42, 6.46 (each d, J=2.5, H–8$_b$ in both moieties), 6.82, 6.88 (each s, H–8 in both moieties), 7.0, 7.08 (each d, J=2.5 H–2 in both moieties)

Aromatic hexahydroxydiphenoyl protons in α- and β- anomers :
6.2, 6.23 (each s, H–2 in both moieties), 6.33, 6.34 (each s, H–2' in both moieties),

Compound (14a):
α-glucose moiety:
5.22 (d, J = 2.5 Hz, H–1–α), 3.75 (m, H–2–α), 5.61 (t, J = 8 Hz, H –3–α), 4.85 (m, H –4– α), 4.45 (m, H –5–α), 5.07 (m, H–6–α), 3.75 (m, H –6'–α).

β-glucose moiety:
4.45 (d, J = 8 Hz, H–1–β ), 3.75 (m, H–2–β), 5.36 (t, J = 8 Hz, H–3–β), 4.85 (m, H–4 – β), 4.48 (m, H–5–β), 5.07 (m, H–6–β), 3.75 (m, H–6'–α) .

Aromatic dehydrodigallicmonocarboxyloyl moiety in α- and β- anomers:

6.39, 6.42 (each d, J=2.5, H–8$_b$ in both moieties), 6.84, 6.88 (each s H–8 in both moieties), 6.95, 7.0 (each d, J =2.5 H–2 in both moieties).

Aromatic hexahydroxydiphenoyl protons in α- and β- anomers :

6.28, 6.3 (each s, H–2 in both moieties), 6.32, 6.35 (each s, H–2' in both moieties).

| | |
|---|---|
| 4. $^{13}$C-NMR Spectral Data<br><br>(DMSO-d$_6$)δ (ppm) | Compound (14):<br><br>glucose moiety:<br>α-anomer:<br>89.5 (C-1), 72.3 (C-2), 70.4 (C-3), 70.3 (C-4), 69.8 (C-5), 62.5 (C-6).<br><br>β-anomer:<br>95.3 (C-1), 72.9 (C-2), 71.5 (C-3), 71.5 (C-4), 65.7 (C-5), 62.5 (C-6).<br><br>galloyl moiety in both anomers:<br>118.4 (C-1), 108.1, 108.9(C-2, C-6), 145.1, 145.2(C-3, C-5) 138.8, 138.9(C-4), 165.3, 165.4 (C=O).<br><br>HHDP moiety in both anomers:<br>123.7, 124.3 (C-1, C-1'), 105.4, 105.6, 105.7 (C-2, C-2') 144.1 (C-3,C-3', C-5, C-5'), 135.3, 135.5 (C-4, C-4'), 115.4, 115.5 (C-6,C-6'), 167.5, 167.6, 167.7 (C=O).<br><br>Dehydrodigalloyl moiety in both anomers:<br>119.6, 120.0 (C-1), 106.7, 107.7 (C-2), 146.5, 146.6 (C-3), 140.1 (C-4), 147.0, 147.1 (C-4$_a$), 112.6,112.7 (C-8$_b$), 136.3, 136.6 (C-4$_b$), 142.2, 142.4 (C-5), 142.2(C-6), 142.4 (C-7), 110.4, 110.6 (C-8), 115.4 (C-8$_a$), 162.3, 162.4 (esterified C=O), 166.9, 167.0 (C=O of free COOH) |

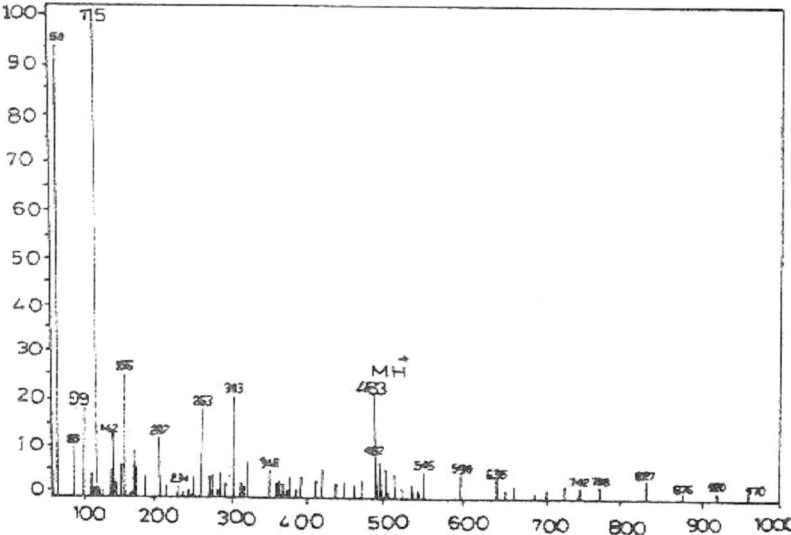

Fig. (37): Positive ESI-MS spectrum of 4, 6-O-hexahydroxybiphenoyl glucose

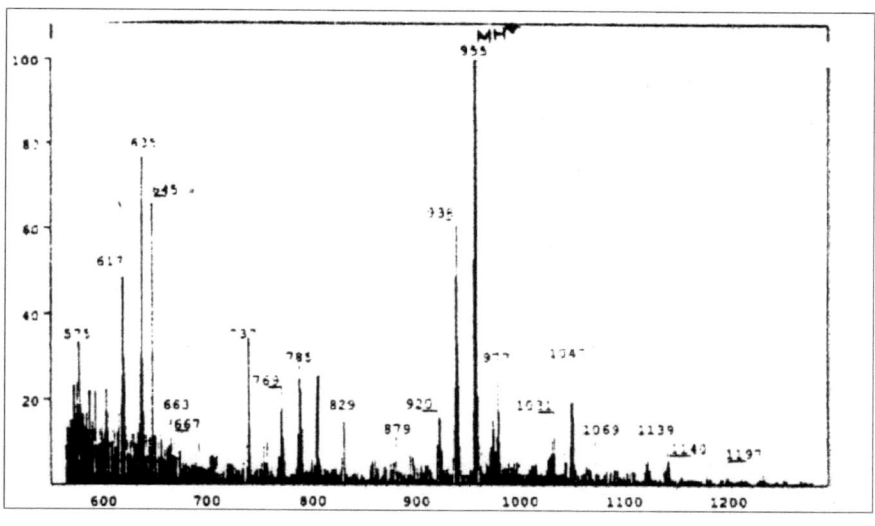

Fig. (38): Positive ESI-MS spectrum of compound (14)

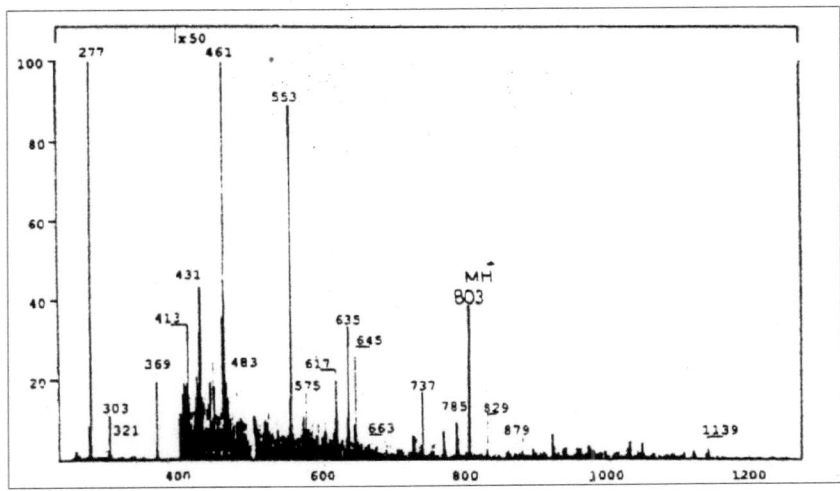

**Fig. (39): Positive ESI-MS spectrum of compound (14a)**

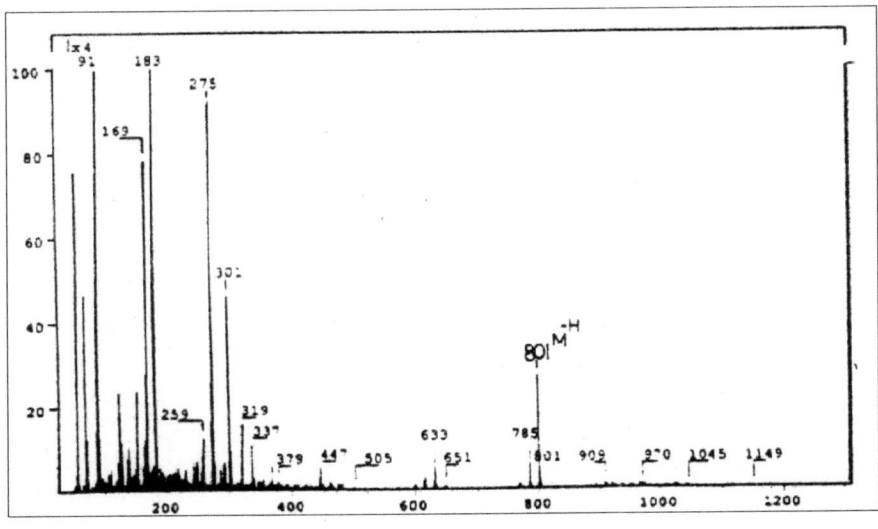

**Fig.(40): Negative ESI-MS spectrum of compound (14a)**

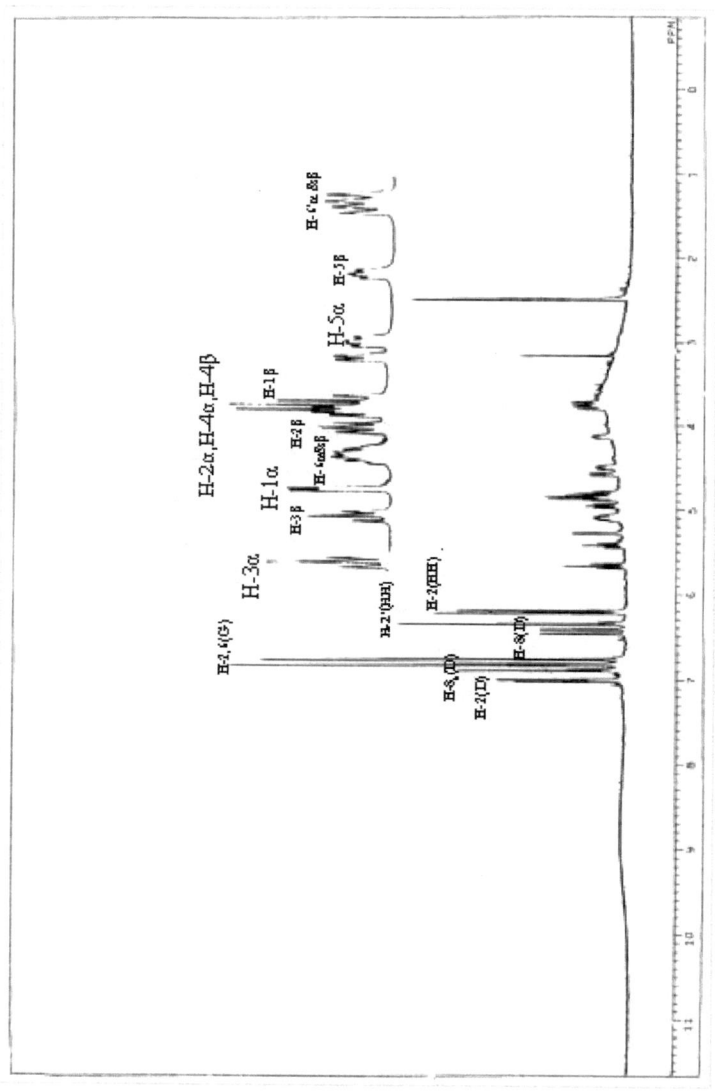

Fig. (41): $^1$H-NMR spectrum of compound (14)

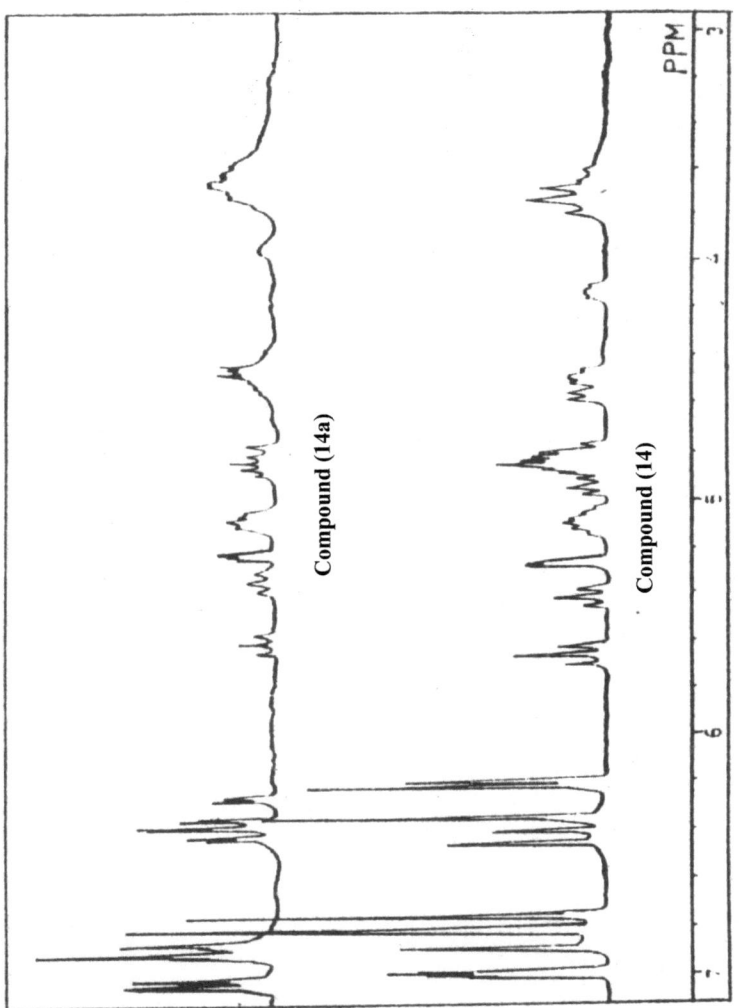

Fig. (42): $^1$H-NMR spectrum of compound (14a)

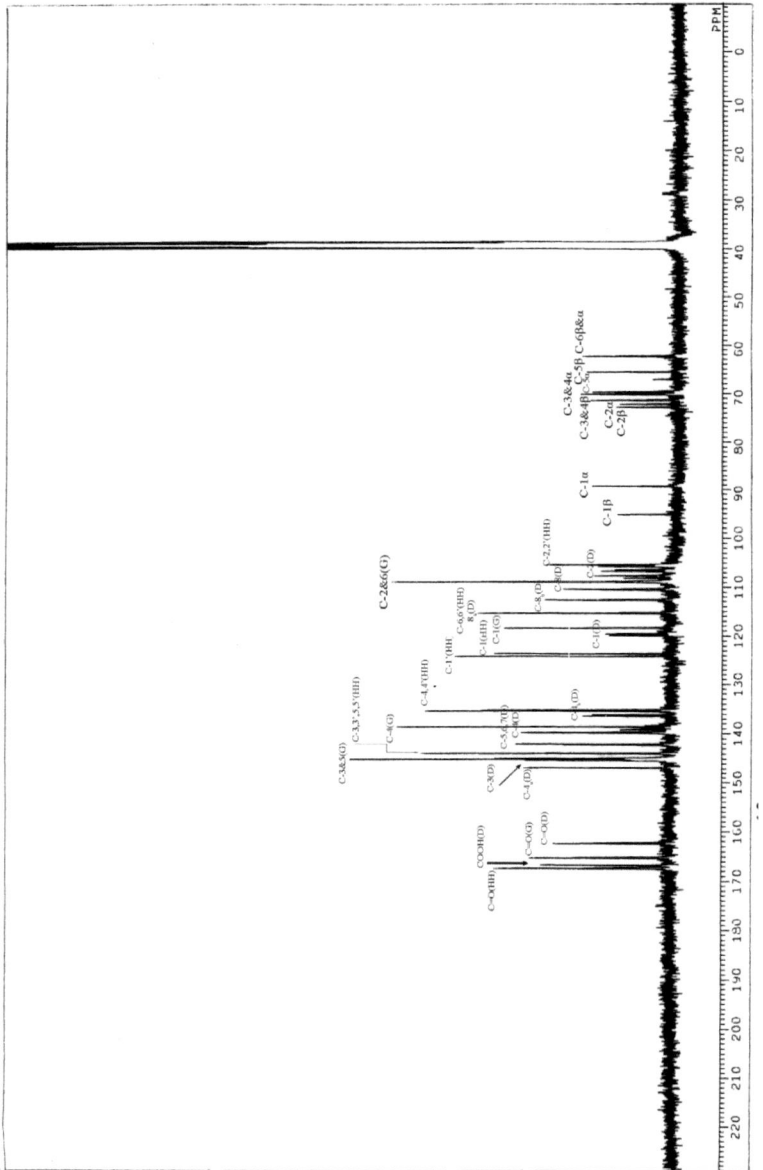

Fig. (43): $^{13}C$ – NMR spectrum of compound (14)

## Fraction X

This fraction showed on 2DPC, a pattern of phenolic spots (deep green colour with $FeCl_3$ spray reagent). However, two major compounds (**15**), and (**16**), exhibited flavonoid characters, and appeared on chromatogram under UV light as dark purple spots turning yellow on fuming with ammonia vapour.

## Isolation of compounds (15) and (16):

Column (45 x 2.5 cm) fractionation of 1.19 g material of fraction X (5.7 g, eluted with 80 % MeOH) over 35 g Sephadex LH-20 using $n$-BuOH saturated with $H_2O$ for elution afforded pure sample of compounds **15** (48 mg) and **16** (37 mg).

## Identification of compound (15): Kaempferol 3-*O*-α-rhamnopyranoside (Afzelin)

Compound **15** (48 mg) was separated as a pale yellow amorphous powder which appeared as a dark purple spot on PC under UV light which changed to lemon yellow on exposure to ammonia vapours. The chromatographic properties and UV spectral data (Table 20) were similar to those reported for kaempferol 3-*O*-α-rhamnoside (Dudek-Makuch and Matawska, 2011) Compound **15** exhibited a molecular weight of 432 in its negative ESI-MS analysis ([M–H]⁻ at $m/z$ =431), (Fig.44).

Complete aqueous acid hydrolysis for 2 hrs over a boiling water bath yielded rhamnose as confirmed by CoPC against authentic sugar markers. The hydrolysis process yielded also an aglycone (**15$_a$**) which was extracted from the aqueous hydrolysate by ethyl acetate, dried under reduced pressure and identified by CoPC, $^1$H-NMR, $^{13}$C-NMR and UV spectral analysis (Table 22) to be kaempferol.

Enzymatic hydrolysis of **15** with α-rhamnosidase (pectinase) in acetate buffer of pH 5.2, at $37°$ C for 24 hrs. was then carried out (Imperato, 1979; Nawwar *et al.*, 1984b). Extraction of the hydrolysate by ethyl acetate and dryness in vacuum followed by CoPC against authentic flavonol samples proved the identity of the released aglycone as kaempferol. The data given above proved kaempferol 3-*O*-α-rhamnoside. Confirmation of this structure was finally achieved through $^1$H-NMR (Fig.45) spectral analysis (Table.20) which revealed the characteristic pattern of proton resonance of kaempferol. Proton resonance in the aromatic region include δ 6.18 ppm (1H, *d, J*=2.5) and 6.38 (1H, *d, J*=2.5) corresponding to H-6 and H-8 respectively. Also, 6.89 (2H, d, *J*=8.4) and 7.7 (2H, d, *J*=8.4 ), are typical of an AX system in

B ring in addition, an anomeric α-rhamnose proton resonance was recognized in this spectrum as a doublet at δppm 5.26 of a coupling constant $J=$ 1.5. In this spectrum, the methyl rhamnose proton resonance revealed itself at 0.77 (d, $J=$ 6). The $^{13}$C-NMR (Fig. 46) spectrum revealed carbon resonances (Table 20), of α-rhamnose moiety, thus finally confirming the identity of compound **15** to be Kaempferol 3-*O*-α-rhamnopyranoside (Song *et al.*, 2007).

**Kaempferol 3-*O*-α-rhamnopyranoside**

**Table (20): Chromatographic and spectral data of aglycone (15)**

| | |
|---|---|
| 1. $R_f$ values (x 100) | 24 ($H_2O$), 47 (AcOH-6), 76 (BAW) |
| 2. UV spectral data $\lambda_{max}$ (nm) | MeOH: 266, 345<br>NaOMe: 271, 376<br>NaOAC: 270, 346<br>NaOAC + $H_3BO_3$ : 270, 346*, 405<br>$Al_3Cl_3$ : 268, 340 *, 385 |
| 3. $^1$H- NMR spectral data (DMSO-$d_6$)δ (ppm) | Kaempferol moiety:<br>6.18 (1H, d, $J=$2.5, H-6)<br>6.38 (1H, d, $J=$2.5, H-8)<br>7.7 (2H, d, $J=$8.4, H-2' and H-6')<br>6.89 (2H, d, $J=$8.4, H-3' and H-5')<br><br>Sugar moiety:<br>5.26 (1H, d, $J=$1.5, H-1")<br>3.4-4.0 (m, sugar protons overlapped with $H_2O$ protons, H2"-5")<br>0.77 (3H, d, $J=$6, H- Me) |

| | |
|---|---|
| 4. $^{13}$C-NMR spectral data (DMSO-$d_6$)δ (ppm) | Keampferol moiety:<br>157.7 (C-2), 134.6 (C-3), 178.14 (C-4), 161.7 (C-5), 99.35 (C-6), 165.19 (C-7), 94.32 (C-8), 157.0 (C-9), 104.4 (C-10), 120.99 (C-1'), 131.1 (C-2' and C-6'), 115.9 (C-3' and C-5'), 160.5 (C-4')<br><br>Sugar moiety:<br>102.2(C-1"), 70.58 (C-2"), 70.79 (C-3"), 71.47 (C-4"), 70.57 (C-5"), 17.97 (C-Me) |

Compound 15a

| | |
|---|---|
| 1. $R_f$ values (x 100) | 0 ($H_2O$), 10 (AcOH-6), 85 (BAW) |
| 2. UV spectral data $\lambda_{max}$ (nm) | MeOH: 268, 369<br>NaOMe : 270, 310, 375<br>NaOAC: 270, 320, 372<br>NaOAC + $H_3BO_3$ : 270, 305*, 360, 430*<br>$Al_3Cl_3$ : 255*, 269, 348, 422 |
| 3. $^1$H- NMR spectral data (DMSO-$d_6$)δ (ppm) | 6.2 (1H, $d$, $J$=2.5, H-6)<br>6.4 (1H, $d$, $J$=2.5, H-8)<br>8.0 (2H, $d$, $J$=8, H-2' and H-6')<br>6.9 (2H, $d$, $J$=8, H-3' and H-5') |
| 4. $^{13}$C-NMR spectral data (DMSO-$d_6$)δ (ppm) | 146.8 (C-2), 135.5 (C-3), 175.9 (C-4), 161.0 (C-5), 98.60 (C-6), 164.2 (C-7), 93.80 (C-8), 156.4 (C-9), 103.7 (C-10), 121.9 (C-1'), 129.9 (C-2' and C-6'), 115.8 (C-3' and C-5'), 159.5 (C-4' |

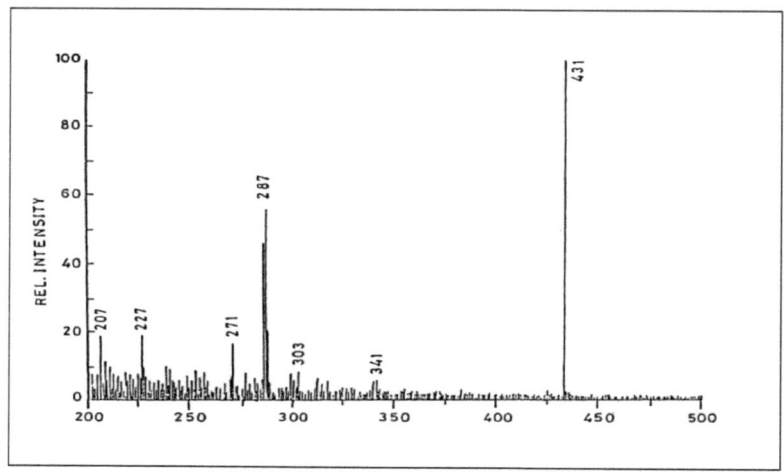

Fig. (44): ESI-MS spectrum of compound (15)

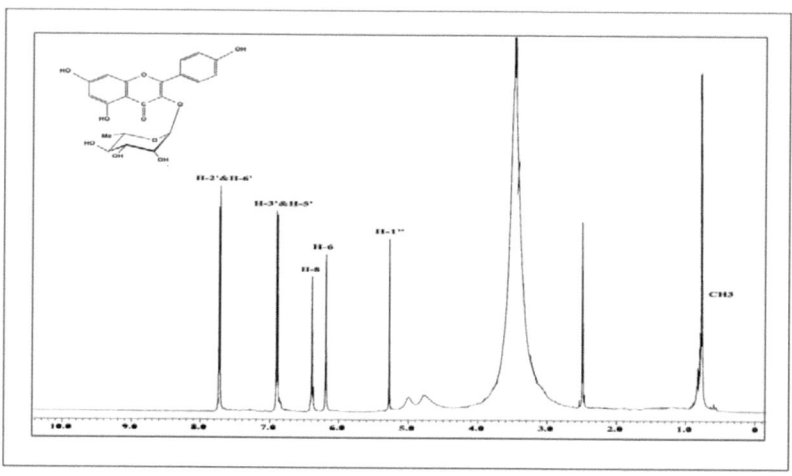

Fig. (45): $^1$H-NMR spectrum of compound (15)

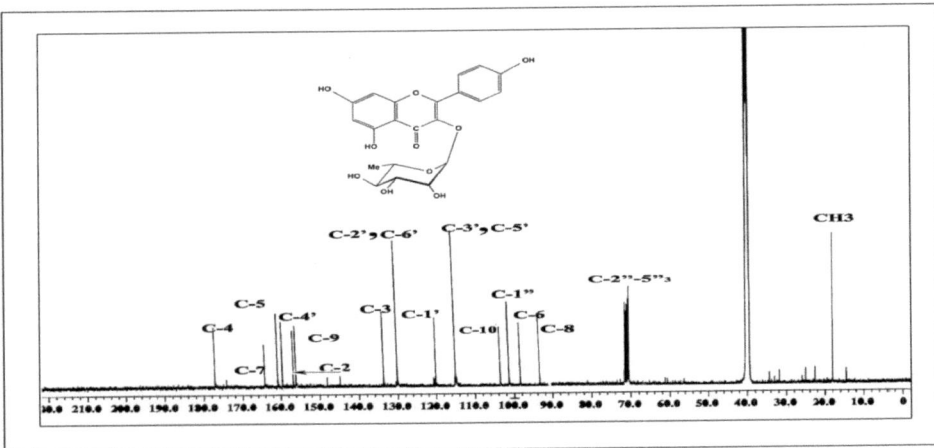

Fig. (46): $^{13}$C-NMR spectrum of compound (15)

## Identification of compound (16): Quercetin 3-$O$-α-rhamnoside

The pure pale yellow amorphous powder of compound **16** (37 mg) has shown chromatographic properties (Table 21), (dark purple spot on paper chromatograms under UV light turning orange when fumed with $NH_3$ vapor or sprayed with Naturstoff specific for flavonoids and giving a green color on spraying with $FeCl_3$). UV absorption maxima in methanol and on the addition of diagnostic shift reagents (Table 21), which were identical with those of an authentic sample of quercetin 3-$O$-α-rhamnoside, quercetrin, which exhibited a $Mr$ of 448 in ESI-MS analysis ([M-H]⁻ at $m/z$ = 447.1), (Fig.47).

Complete aqueous acid hydrolysis for 2 hours over a boiling water bath yielded rhamnose as was confirmed by CoPC against authentic sugar markers. The hydrolysis process yielded as well an aglycone **16a**, which was extracted from the aqueous hydrolysate by ethyl acetate, dried under reduced pressure and identified by CoPC and UV spectral analysis to be quercetin.

Enzymatic hydrolysis of **16** with α-rhamnosidase (pectinase) (Nawwar et al., 1984b) in acetate buffer of pH 5.2, at 37° C for 24 hours was then performed. Extraction of the hydrolysate by ethyl acetate and dryness in vacuum followed by CoPC against authentic flavonol samples proved the identity of the released aglycone as quercetin.

From the above given data, compound **16** was therefore, proved to be quercetin 3-$O$-α-rhamnoside, quercitrin (Takeya and Itokawa, 1988). Confirmation of the proposed structure of **16** was achieved through $^1$H-NMR spectroscopic analysis. The recorded spectrum (DMSO-$d_6$, room temperature), (Fig.48) revealed in the aromatic region the characteristic pattern of quercetin proton resonances (Table 21). In addition, the spectrum revealed also an anomeric proton resonance, appearing as a broad singlet of $\Delta v_{1/2}$ = 4 Hz, at δ 5.2 ppm assignable to the rhamnoside proton $H^{-1}$. This measured half-line width proved the α-configuration at the anomeric rhamnoside carbon and proved therefore, the $^1C_4$-conformation of this moiety.

Final confirmation of the identity was achieved through $^{13}$C-NMR spectroscopic analysis of **16**. In the received spectrum (DMSO-$d_6$, room temperature), (Fig. 49), the presence of a rhamnose moiety followed from the signal of the aliphatic methyl carbon at δ 18.01 ppm. The signal of the C-3 carbon of the flavonol moiety at δppm 134.6 showed the direct bonding between both sugar and aglycone moieties at the flavonol C-3 position (Table 21).

Consequently, component **16** is identified to be quercetin 3-$O$-$\alpha$-$^1C_4$-rhamnopyranoside or quercitrin (Takeya and Itokawa, 1988).

**Quercetin 3-$O$-$\alpha$-rhamnoside**

**Table (21): Chromatographic and spectral data of compound (16)**

| 1. $R_f$ values (x 100) | 22 ($H_2O$), 48 (AcOH-6), 68 (BAW) |
|---|---|
| 2. UV spectral data $\lambda_{max}$ (nm) | MeOH: 259, 297 sh., 348<br>NaOMe: 270, 355, 402<br>NaOAC: 276, 372<br>NaOAC + $H_3BO_3$: 272, 383<br>Al $Cl_3$ : 268, 352, 408 |
| 3. $^1$H- NMR spectral data (DMSO-$d_6$)$\delta$ (ppm) | Quercetin moiety:<br>6.17 (1H, $d$, $J$=2.5 Hz, H-6),<br>6.36 (1H, $d$, $J$=2.5 Hz, H-8),<br>7.256 (1H, $d$, $J$=2.5, H-2'),<br>6.82 (1H, $d$, $J$=8 Hz, H-5'),<br>7.251 (1H, $dd$, $J$=2.5 and 8 Hz, H-6')<br><br>Rhamnose moiety:<br>5.20 (1H, $\Delta v_{1/2}$= 4 Hz, H-1"),<br>3.1 – 3.9 ($m$, overlapped with water proton resonances, H-2"-H-6") |

| | |
|---|---|
| 4. $^{13}$C-NMR spectral data (DMSO-$d_6$)δ (ppm) | Quercetin moiety:<br>156.9 (C-2), 134.6 (C-3), 178.2 (C-4), 161.7(C-5), 99.19 (C-6), 164.7 (C-7), 94.15(C-8), 157.8 (C-9), 104.5 (C-10),121.2 (C-1'),115.9 (C-2'), 145.7 (C-3'), 148.9(C-4'), 116.1(C-5'), 121.6 (C-6')<br><br>Rhamnose moiety:<br>102.2 (C-1"), 70.8 (C-2"), 71.1 (C-3"), 71.6 (C-4"), 70.5 (C-5"), 18.01(CH$_3$). |

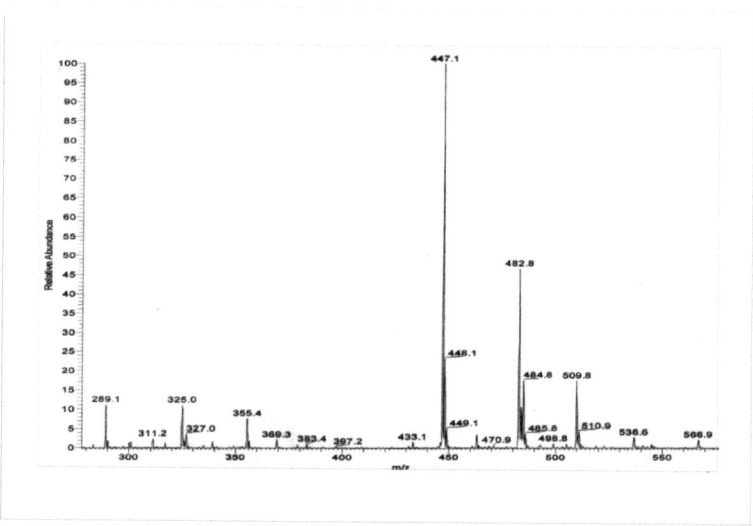

Fig. (47): Negative ESI/MS spectrum of compound (16)

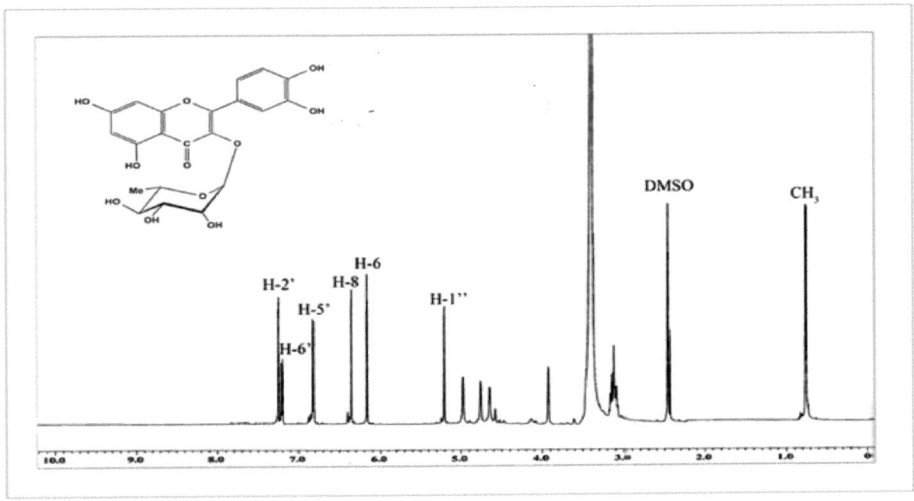

Fig. (48): $^1$H- NMR spectrum of compound (16)

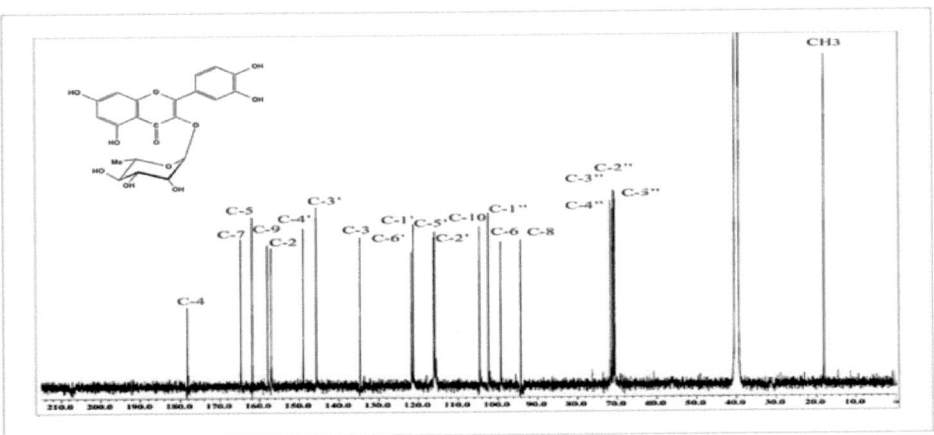

Fig. (49): $^{13}$C- NMR spectrum of compound (16)

## Fraction XI

This fraction showed on 2DPC four major components **(17)**, **(17∗)**, **(18)** and **(19)** which appeared as yellow spots under UV light and gave positive $FeCl_3$ test.

## Isolation of compounds (17), (17*) (18), (19)

Compounds **17** (49 mg), (**17∗** 25 mg), **18** (38 mg) and, **19** (19 mg) were individually isolated from 792 mg of the major column fraction XI (3.4 g, eluted by 90 % MeOH) through repeated prep. PC using BAW as solvent.

## Identification of compound (17): Kaempferol

Compound **17** was obtained as yellow amorphous powder (49 mg) and appeared as a yellow spot on PC under UV light, which changed lemon yellow on exposure to $NH_3$. UV spectral data (Table 22) and a *Mr* of 286 in its negative ESI-MS analysis ([M-H]⁻ at *m/z* =285) (Fig. 50) suggests that compound **17** was the aglycone kaempferol. The $^1$H-NMR spectral data (Fig. 51) (Table 22) was found to be in accordance with the proposed structure. Also, CoPC with authentic kaempferol confirmed the identity (Harborne, 1982)

**Compound (17): Kaempferol**

## Table (22): Chromatographic and spectral data of compound (17)

| | |
|---|---|
| 1. $R_f$ values (x 100) | 00 ($H_2O$), 10 (HOAc-6), 85 (BAW) |
| 2. UV Spectral Data $\lambda_{max}$ (nm), MeOH | MeOH (a): 268, 369; NaOAc (b):270, 310, 375; $H_3BO_3$ : 270, 320, 372; $AlCl_3$ (c) :270, 305, 360, 430; HCl :255, 269, 348, 422; MeONa :278, 316, 413. |
| 3. $^1$H-NMR Spectral Data (DMSO-$d_6$) δ (ppm) | 6.4 (d, J=2.5, H-8), 6.18 (d, J=2.5, H-6) 8.14 (d., J=8, H-2' and H-6'), 6.89 (d, J=8, H-3' and H-5'). |

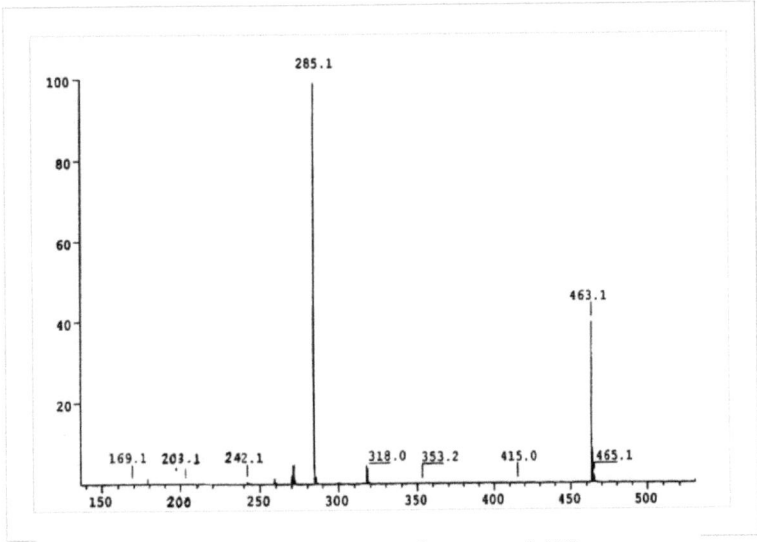

Fig. (50): ESI -MS spectrum of compound (17)

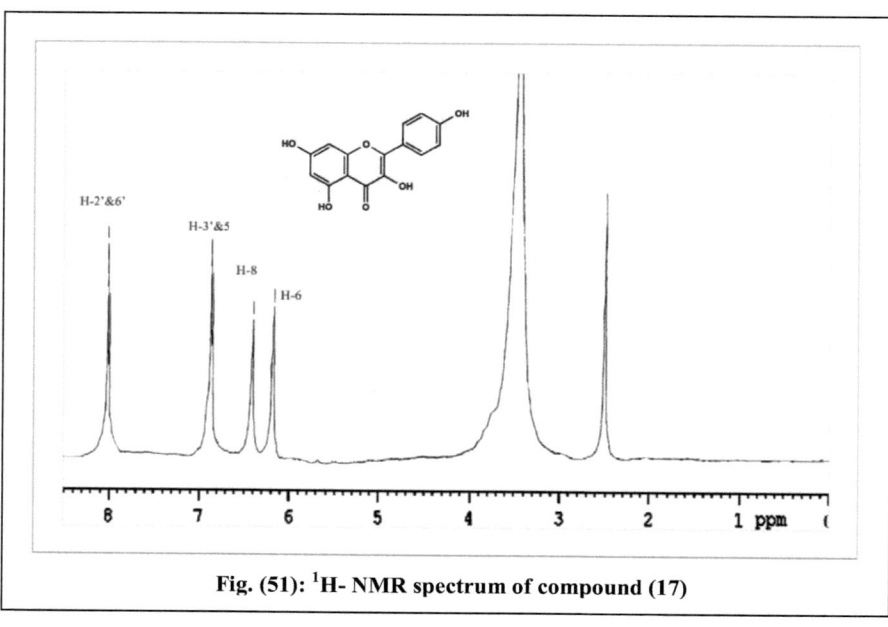

Fig. (51): $^1$H- NMR spectrum of compound (17)

## Identification of compound (17∗): Kaempheride

Compound (17) was obtained as yellow amorphous powder (25 mg) and appeared as a yellow spot on PC under UV light, which changed lemon yellow on exposure to $NH_3$. UV spectral data (Table 23) and a $Mr$ of 286 in its negative ESI-MS analysis ([M-H]⁻ at $m/z$ =285) suggests that compound (15) was the aglycone kaempheride. The $^1$H-NMR spectral data (Fig. 52) (Table 23) was found to be in accordance with the proposed structure. Also, CoPC with authentic kaempheride confirmed the identity (Harborne, 1982). Final confirmation of the identity was achieved through $^{13}$C-NMR spectroscopic analysis of **17∗**(Fig. 53) (Table 23).

**Compound (17): Kaempheride**

**Table (23): Chromatographic and spectral data of compound (17∗)**

| | | Kaempferide: |
|---|---|---|
| 1. | $R_f$ values (x 100) | 0.92 (BAW) |
| 2. | UV Spectral Data $\lambda_{max}$ (nm),MeOH | MeOH: 267, 300 shoulder, 367; NaOMe: 280, 404; NaOAc: 272, 310, 384; NaOAc-$H_3BO_3$: 267, 300 shoulder, 364; $AlCl_3$: 270, 304, 345, 420 shoulder; 367. |
| 3. | ESIMS (negative mode), $m/z$: | 286 |
| 4. | $^1$H- NMR spectral data (DMSO-$d_6$)δ (ppm) | 8.15 (2H, d, J = 8.5 Hz, H-2' and H-6'), 7.05 (2H, d, J=8.5 Hz, H-3' and H-5'), 6.45 (1H, d, J=2 Hz, H-8); 6.20 (1H, d, J=2 Hz, H-6). |
| 5. | $^{13}$C-NMR spectral data (DMSO-$d_6$)δ (ppm) | 146.7 (C-2), 135.7 (C-3), 175.9 (C-4), 160.7 (C-5), 98.2 (C-6), 163.9 (C-7), 93.5 (C-8), 156.2 (C-9), 103.0 (C-10), 123.2 (C-1'), 129.5 (C-2' & C-6'), 114.2 (C-3' & C-5'), 160.2 (C-4'), 55.9 (C-4'OMe) |

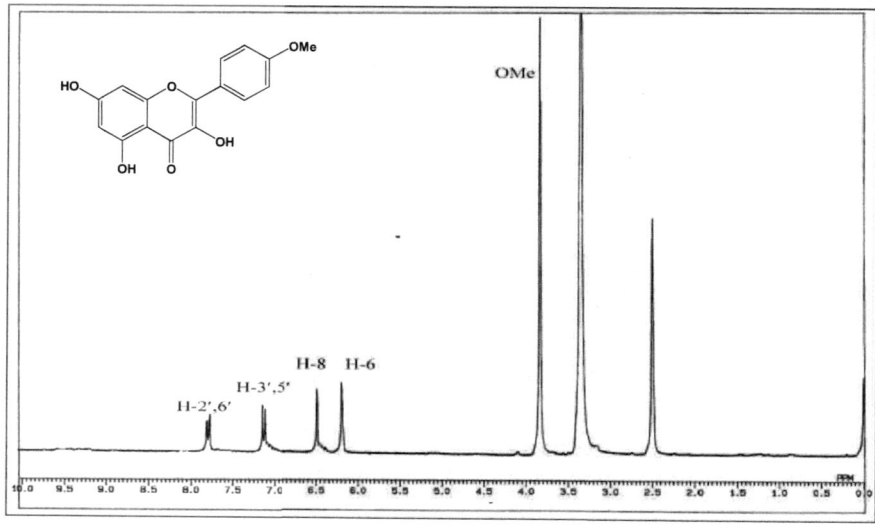

Fig. (52): $^1$H- NMR spectrum of compound (17∗)

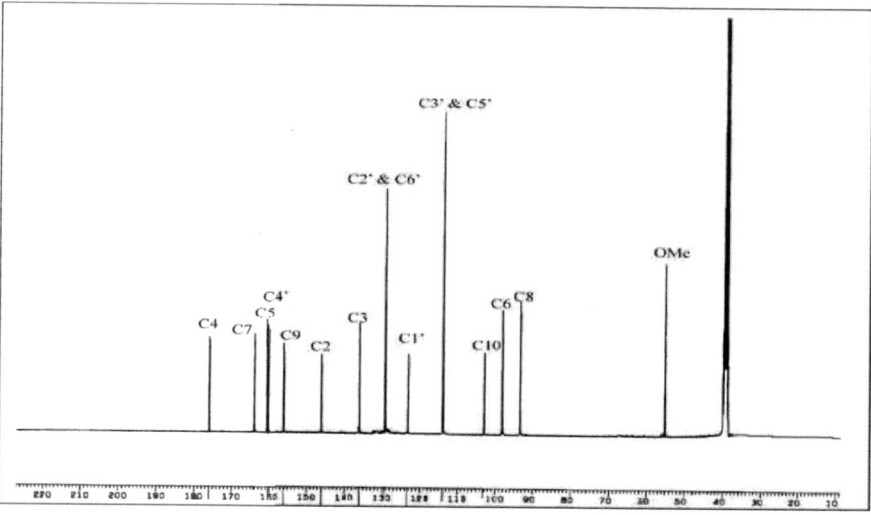

Fig. (53): $^{13}$C- NMR spectrum of compound (17∗)

## Identification of compound (18): Tamarixetin

Compound **18** was obtained as yellow amorphous powder (38 mg) and appeared as a yellow spot on PC under UV light, which changed to dull yellow on exposure to $NH_3$ vapors and UV spectral data (Table 24).

The $^1$H-NMR (Fig. 54) and $^{13}$C-NMR (Fig. 55) spectral data (Table 24) was found to be in agreement with the proposed structure and suggest that compound **18** was the aglycone tamarixetin. The identity of compound **18** was further confirmed by UV and CoPC with an authentic sample (Urbatsch *et al.*, 1976).

**Compound (18): Tamarixetin**

## Table (24): Chromatographic and spectral data of compounds (18)

| | | |
|---|---|---|
| 1. | $R_f$ values (x 100) | 8 ($H_2O$), 17 (HOAc-6), 83 (BAW) |
| 2. | UV Spectral Data $\lambda_{max}$ (nm), MeOH | MeOH: 238, 255, 268, 369;<br>NaOMe: 268, 422;<br>NaOAC: 253 (inflection), 273, 312, 360 sh.;<br>NaOAc - $H_3BO_3$: 255, 265 inf., 368;<br>$AlCl_3$: 268, 301 inf., 363, 430;<br>$AlCl_3$ + HCl: 268, 301 inf., 362, 426. |
| 3. | $^1$H- NMR Spectral Data (DMSO-$d_6$)$\delta$ (ppm) | 6.22 (1H, $d$, $J$= 2 Hz, H-6),<br>6.45 (1H, $d$, $J$=2 Hz, H-8),<br>7.08 (1H, $d$, $J$ =8 Hz, H-5'),<br>7.65 (m, H-2' and H-6'),<br>3.81 ($s$, Me-4'). |
| 4. | $^{13}$C-NMR Spectral Data (DMSO-$d_6$)$\delta$ (ppm) | 146.2 (C – 2), 136 (C – 3), 175.9 (C – 4), 160.8 (C – 5), 98 (C – 6), 163.9 (C – 7), 93.3 (C – 8), 156.2 (C – 9), 103 (C – 10), 123.2 (C – 1'), 114.80 (C - 2'), 146 (C – 3'), 149.01 (C – 4'), 111.50 (C – 5'), 119.40 (C – 6'), 55.8 ( Me-4'). |

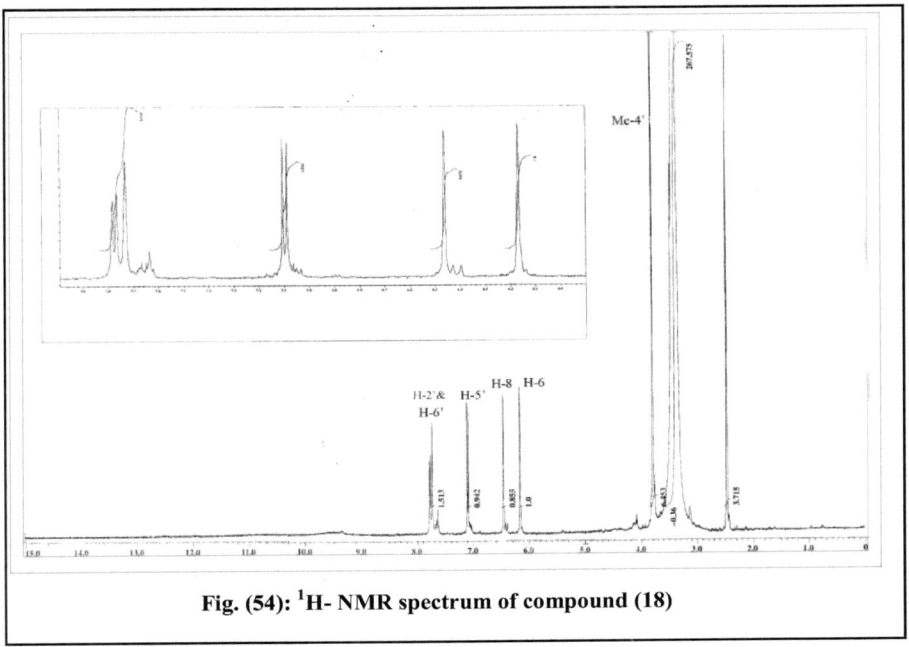

Fig. (54): $^1$H- NMR spectrum of compound (18)

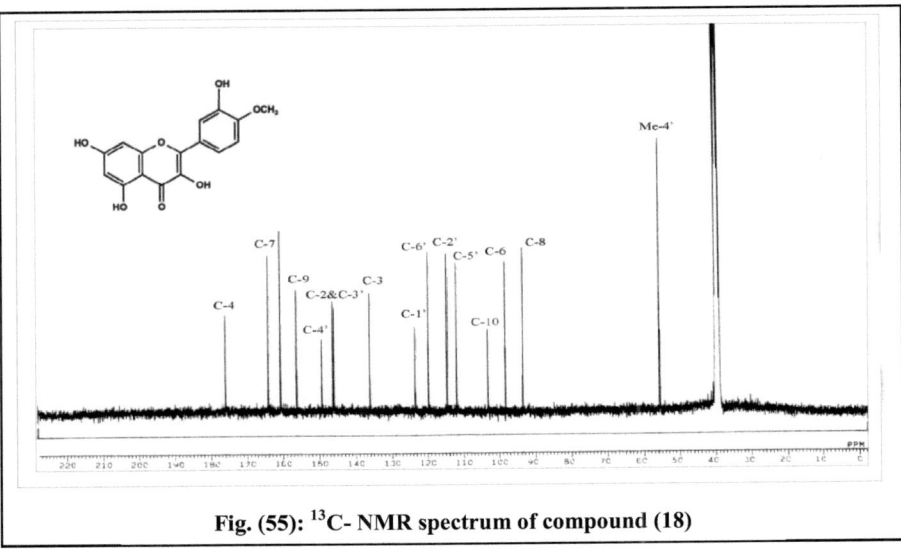

Fig. (55): $^{13}$C- NMR spectrum of compound (18)

## Identification of compound (19): Quercetin

Compound **19** was obtained as yellow amorphous powder (19 mg) and appeared as a yellow spot on PC under UV light, which changed orange on exposure to $NH_3$ vapors, UV spectral data (Table 25) and a $Mr$ of 302 in its negative ESI-MS analysis ([M-H]⁻ at $m/z$ =301) (Fig. 56) suggests that compound 17 is possibly quercetin.

The $^1$H-NMR (Fig. 57) (Table 25) spectral data was found to be in accordance with the proposed structure. The identity of compound **19** was further confirmed by CoPC with an authentic sample as well as comparing the spectral data for those reported for quercetin (Harborne, 1982).

**Compound (19): Quercetin**

**Table (25): Chromatographic and spectral data of compound (19)**

| | |
|---|---|
| 1. $R_f$ values (x 100) | 00 ($H_2O$), 07 (HOAc-6), 75 (BAW) |
| 2. UV Spectral Data $\lambda_{max}$ (nm), MeOH | MeOH : 255, 268, 370;<br>NaOAc : 254, 276, 375;<br>$H_3BO_3$ : 272, 388;<br>$AlCl_3$ : 270, 360, 440;<br>$AlCl_3$+ HCl : 258, 400. |
| 3. $^1$H- NMR Spectral Data (DMSO-$d_6$)δ (ppm) | 6.19 ($d$, $J$=2.5, H-6), 6.4 ($d$, $J$=2.5, H-8), 7.64 ($d$, $J$=2.5, H-2'), 6.88 ($d$, $J$=8.5, H-5'), 7.53 ($dd$, $J$=2.5&8.5, H-6'). |

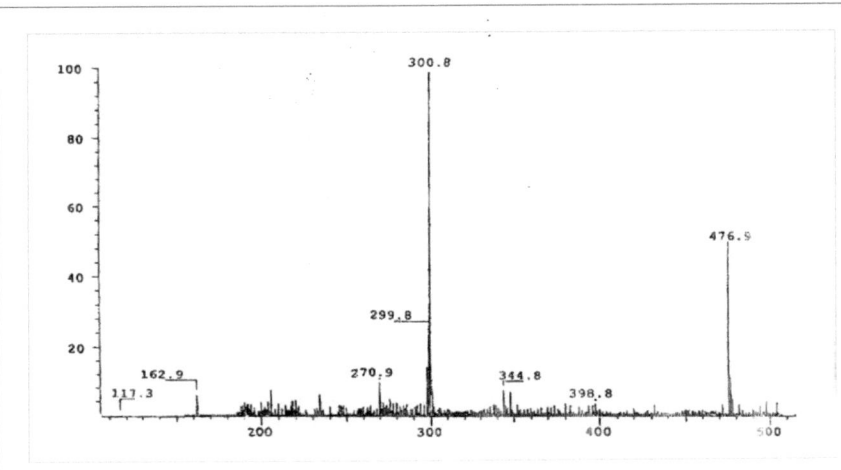

Fig. (56): ESI-MS spectrum of compound (19)

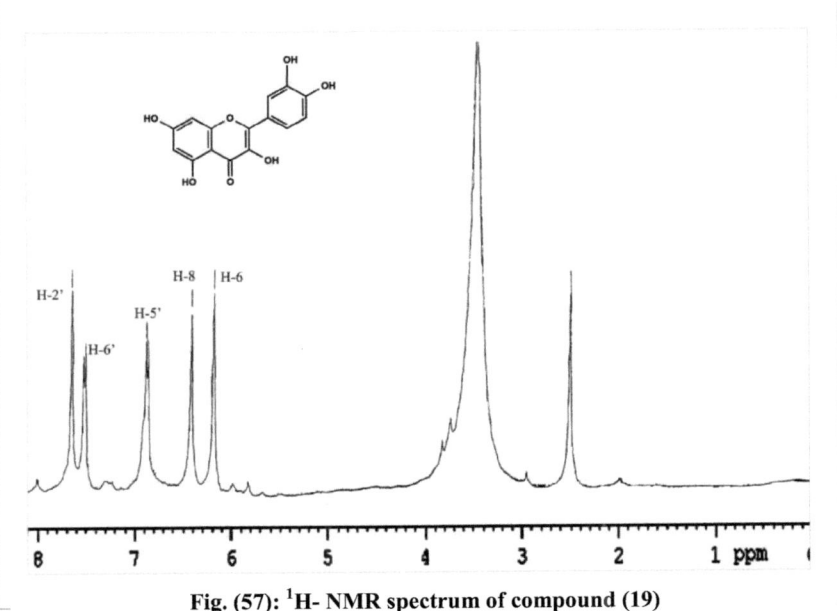

Fig. (57): $^1$H- NMR spectrum of compound (19)

## Fraction XII

2DPC of this fraction showed one single spot compound (**20**). It appeared with mauve color under UV, which turned yellow when fumed with ammonia and gave positive reaction with Ninhydrin and $FeCl_3$.

## Isolation of compound (20)

Compound **20** was separated pure from fraction XII (2DPC). Removal of the solvent under reduced pressure at 40°C afforded an oil sample of **20** (112 mg).

## Identification of compound (20): *N-trans*-3-Hydroxy 4-methoxy cinnamoyltyramine, (Tamgermanetin)

Compound **20** (112 mg), isolated as pale yellow oil, which gave a positive reaction with ninhydrin and phenol reagent. Spots of **20** on PC appeared with mauve colour, which turned yellow when fumed with ammonia. It was analyzed for the molecular formula $C_{18}H_{19}O_4N$ on the basis of $^1H$, $^{13}C$-NMR and HRESIMS ([M - H]⁻: 312.1203, calc.: 312.3495) (Fig.58&59). IR absorbance bands recorded for **20** at $v_{max}$ (KBr) $cm^{-1}$: 1204, 1430 (C-N stretching), 1625 (-C = O), 2921, 3015 (N-H stretching), 3120 and 3625 $cm^{-1}$ thus proving the presence of hydroxyl and amide carboxyl. The compound presented UV absorption in MeOH at $\lambda_{max}$ 295, 315 nm, which were reminiscent of a phenyl propanoid system. **20** yielded isoferulic acid (mauve color spot on PC which turned yellow when fumed with ammonia, CoPC, $^1H$ and $^{13}C$-NMR) and tyramine hydrocloride (EI-MS, UVabsorption and $^1H$ NMR) on acid hydrolysis [2 N aqueous / methanolic (1:1), HCl, 3 hours, 100°C] (Table26).

$^1$H-NMR spectrum of **20** (Fig. 60) displayed a pair of doublets, each of $J$ = 16 Hz, at δ ppm 6.26 and 7.52 ppm attributable to *trans*-olefinic protons and a distinct set of aromatic protons together with a methoxyl signals assignable to the 3-hydroxy-4-methoxyphenyl moiety of isoferulic acid [δ ppm 7.06 (1H, *d, J*=2 Hz, H-2); 7.05 (1H, *dd, J*=2 Hz and J=8 Hz, H-6); 6.92 (1H, *d, J*=8 Hz, H-5); 3.87 (s, 3H, OMe-3)]. The spectrum also exhibited a second distinct set consisting of a pair of aromatic proton resonances, each integrated to two equivalent protons, and two $sp^3$ methylenic signals all belonging to a phenethyl moiety at δ 6.68 (2H, *d, J*=8 Hz, H-3' and H-5'); 7.04 (2H, *d, J*=8 Hz, H-2' and H-6'); 3.48 (m, 2H, H-8'); 2.54 (1H, *t, J*= 7.3 Hz H-7'). The $^{13}C$-spectrum of **20** (Fig. 13) contained 18 lines , and the DEPT spectrum established the presence of one carbonyl, three quaternary $sp^2$, nine protonated $sp^2$ carbons, and three oxygenated $sp^2$ carbons together with two $sp^3$ methylenic carbons and one $sp^3$ oxygenated methyl carbon. Direct correlation observed in the $^1H$-$^1H$ COSY (Fig 62&63), HSQC and HMBC spectra of **20** allowed unambiguous assignment of protons, protonated and quaternary carbons (Table 26). Analysis of $^1H$-$^1H$ COSY NMR spectroscopic data allowed –$CH_2$-$CH_2$- and CH=CH- subunits to be defined. The connectivity between the protons of these subunits with carbons in the 4-hydroxyphenyl and the carbons of the 3-hydroxy 4-methoxy phenyl moieties was demonstrated by interpretation of the HMBC correlation data. The observed $^3J$ correlations in this spectrum showed that proton H-8' (δ 3.48) correlates to the carbonyl carbon C-9 (δ 165.9) and to the quaternary *p*-hydroxyphenyl C-1' carbon (δ 129.95). Among the $^3J$ correlations recognized one was found correlating the methoxyl proton signal at (δ 3.87) to the aromatic carbon C-4 at (δ 150.7), another correlated the olefinic proton H-7 at (δ 7.52) to carbons C-2 at (δ 113.26), C-6 at (121.57) and to the carbonyl carbon C-9 at 1265.90 and a third correlated the *sp3* methylenic protons 2H-8'at (δ 3.48) to the carbonyl carbon C-9 at (δ165.90), and to the phenethyl carbons (C-1') at δ 129.95. The recognizable $^2J$ correlations recorded in this spectrum (see Experimental) were in accordance with the achieved structure. These and the above given data finally confirmed the structure of compound **20** to be *N-trans*-3-hydroxy 4-methoxy cinnamoyltyramine, for which we give the name tamgermanetin, a unique isoferuloyl derivative. Tamgermanitin (20) is of special interest as it represents the first reported natural occurrence of an isoferulic acid amide. The analogs amide of the positional isomer, ferulic acid has been characterized before, from *Achyranthes bidentata* (Yang et al., 2012) and *Solanum tuberosum* (King and Calhoun, 2005).

**Compound (20): Tamgermanetin (*N-trans*-3-Hydroxy 4-methoxy cinnamoyltyramine)**

**Table (26): Chromatographic and spectral data of compounds (20)**

| | Compound (20) |
|---|---|
| 1. $R_f$ values (x 100) | 0.10 ($H_2O$), 0.19 (AcOH-6), 94 (BAW) |
| 2. UV spectral data $\lambda_{max}$ (nm) (MeOH) | 220, 295, 315 |
| 3. ESI-MS, (negative mode), $m/z$<br>HRESI-MS: $m/z$: | 312, $[M-H]^-$<br>312.1203, calc.: 312.3495 for $C_{18}H_{19}O_4N$ |
| 4. IR absorbance bands $\nu_{max}$ (KBr) cm$^{-1}$ | 1204, 1430 (C-N stretching), 1625 (-C = O), 2921, 3015 (N-H stretching), 3120 and 3625 cm$^{-1}$ |
| 5. $^1$H- NMR spectral data $(CD_3)_2CO$ $\delta$ (ppm) | 7.52 (1H, $d$, $J$ = 16 Hz, H-7), 7.07 (1H, $d$, $J$ = 2.0 Hz, H-2), 7.05 (1H, $dd$, $J$ = 8 Hz, and 2 Hz, H-6), 7.04 (2H, $d$, $J$ = 8 Hz, H-2' and H-6'), 6.92 (1H, $d$, $J$ = 8.0 Hz, H-5), 6.68 (2H, $d$, $J$ = 8 Hz, H-3'and H-5'), 6.26 (1H, $d$, $J$ = 16 Hz, H-8), 3.87 (3H, s, OMe-4), 3.48 (2 H, m, H-8'), 2.54 (2H, $t$, $J$ = 7.7 Hz, H-7'). |
| 6. $^{13}$C-NMR spectral data (DMSO-$d_6$)$\delta$ (ppm) | Isoferuloyl moiety:<br>129.96 (C-1), 113.62 (C-2), 146.90 (C-3), 150.07 (C-4), 115.82 (5), 121.57 (C-6), 139.41 (C-7), 115.84 (C-8), 168.42 (C = O), 55.44 (OMe-4);<br>Tyramine moiety:<br>129.95 (C-1'), 129.99 (C-2' and C-6'), 113.62 (C-3' and C-5'), 156.07 (C-4'), 34.77 (C-7'). 40.17 (C-8'). |

|  | Isoferulic acid: |
|---|---|
| 1. $R_f$ values (x 100) | |
| 2. UV spectral data $\lambda_{max}$ | 37($H_2O$), 45(AcOH-6), 92(BAW) |
| (nm) (MeOH) | 240, 295, 325 |
| 3. $^1$H- NMR spectral data (CD$_3$)$_2$CO) δ (ppm) | 7.51 (1H, d, J = 16 Hz, H-7), 7.13 (1H, d, J = 2 Hz, H – 2), 7.06 (1H, dd, J = 2 Hz and J = 8 Hz, H6), 6.93 (1 H, d, J = 8 Hz, H – 5), 6.26 (1H, d, J = 16 Hz, H – 8) |
| 4. $^{13}$C-NMR spectral data (DMSO-$d_6$)δ (ppm) | 127.2 (C-1), 113.62 (C-2), 146.91 (C-3), 150.70 (C-4), 109.15 (5), 121.57 (C-6), 145.01 (C-7), 115.82 (C-8), 168.43 (C = O) |
|  | Tyramine hydrochloride : |
| 1. UV spectral data λmax (nm) MeOH | 276, 282 |
| 2. EI MS, m/z: | 137 [M]$^+$, 107 (M-CH2NH2), 91, 78, 77, 44, 30 |
| 3. $^1$H- NMR spectral data (D$_2$O) δ (ppm) | 2.9 (2H, t, J =7 Hz), 3.2 (2H, t, J =7 Hz), 6.85 (2H, d, J =8 Hz), 7.2 (2H, d, J =8 Hz) |

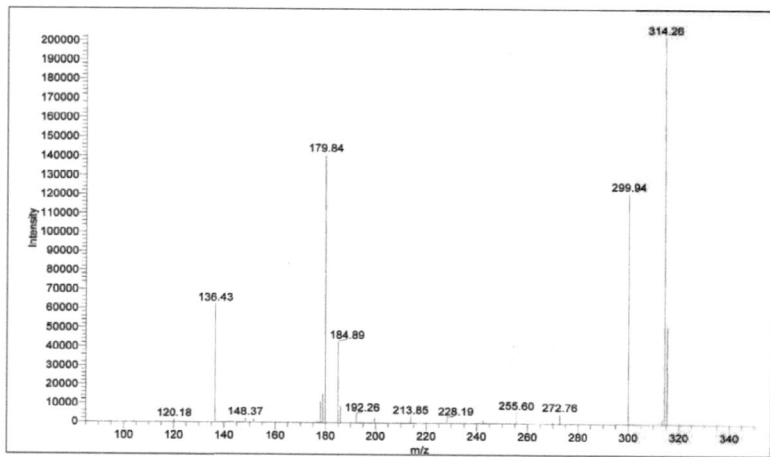

**Fig. (58): Positive ESI-MS of compound (20)**

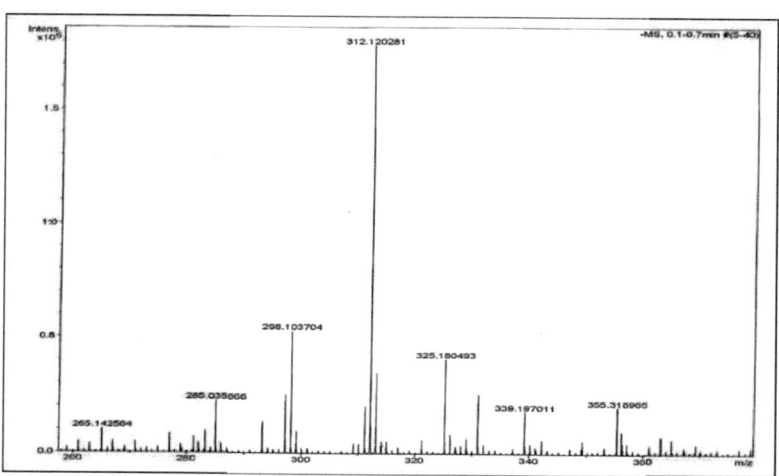

**Fig. (59): Negative ESI-MS of compound (20)**

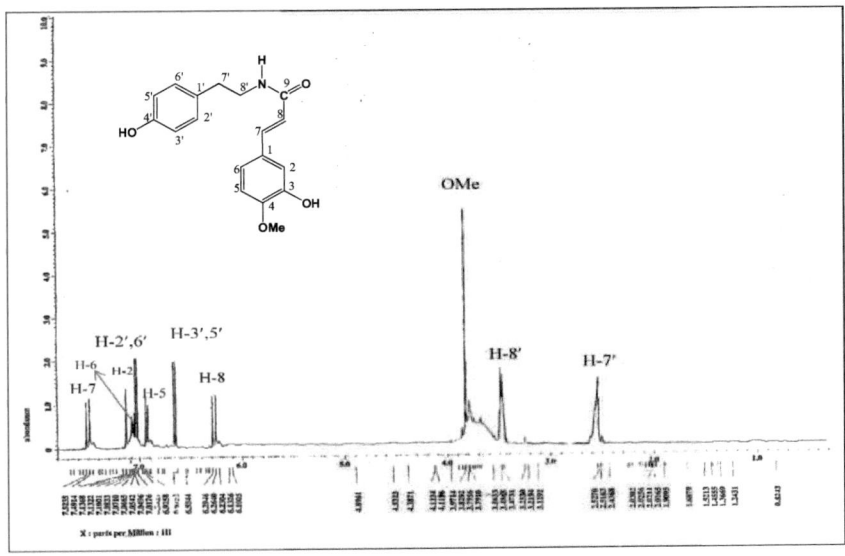

Fig. (60): $^1$H-NMR spectrum of compound (20)

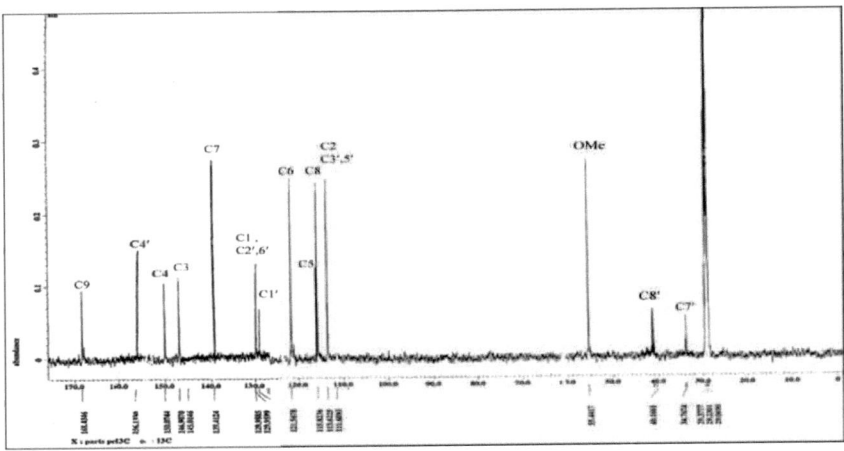

Fig. (61): $^{13}$C-NMR spectrum of compound (20)

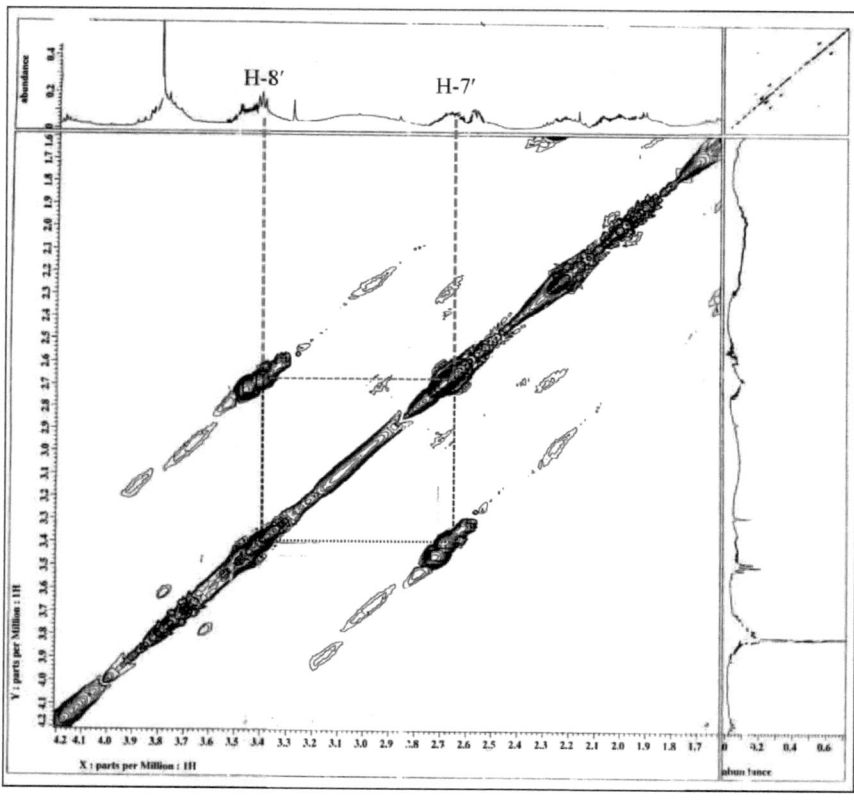

Fig. (62): $^1$H-$^1$H COSY spectrum of aliphatic protons of compound (20)

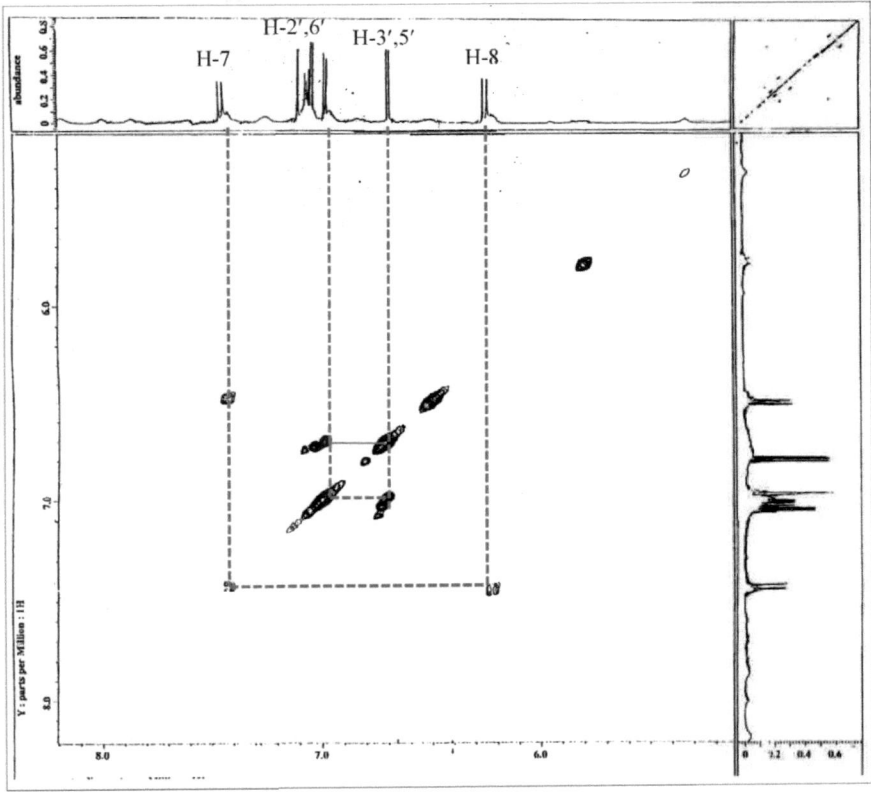

**Fig. (63):** $^1$H-$^1$H COSY spectrum of aromatic protons of compound (20)

# 5. BIOLOGICAL INVESTIGATION OF *Myricaria germanica* AERIAL PARTS EXTRACT, COLUMN FRACTIONS AND ISOLATED COMPOUNDS

## 5.1. Cytotoxicity assessment

SRB-U (Skehan *et al.*, 1990) assay was used to assess the cytotoxicity of the crude extract, column fractions and isolated compounds from *Myricaria germanica* (L.) Desv. against three different tumor cell lines over concentration range 0.01–100 µg/ml. Doxorubicin was used as a positive control. The crude extract per se showed considerable potency against PC-3, Huh-7 and MCF-7 cell lines with $IC_{50}$ values of 6.5, 2.85 and 0.2 µg/ml, respectively. MCF-7 cell line showed relatively high resistance fraction (R-value) after treatment with the crude extract with resistance fraction of 8.4% while there were negligible R-values for PC-3 and Huh-7 cells (0 and 0.55%, respectively).

Tamarixellagic acid showed the most potent cytotoxicity against PC-3 prostate cancer cell line ($IC_{50}$ = 0.13 µg/ml) with 0.0% resistance fraction; the other column fractions showed less potent cytotoxic effects with $IC_{50}$'s ranging from 0.22 to 6.2 µg/ml.

In Huh 7 liver cancer cell line, column fractions IV (gallic acid and 3-methoxygallic acid) and tamarixellagic acid showed the most potent cytotoxic profile with $IC_{50}$ of 0.03 µg/ml for both fractions with R-value of 3.7% and 5.9%, respectively. Other column fractions showed much lower but considerable cytotoxic profile against Huh-7 cell line with $IC_{50}$ values ranging from 0.13–11.5 µg/ml.

In case of MCF-7 breast cancer cell line, column fraction IV (gallic acid and 3-methoxygallic acid), 2,6-di-*O*- galloyl-($\alpha/\beta$)-glucose and tamarixellagic acid showed the highest cytotoxic profile with $IC_{50}$'s of 0.13 µg/ml, 0.15 µg/ml and 0.16 µg/ml, respectively and the resistance fraction was 0.0%. The other fractions showed milder but considerable cytotoxic effect with $IC_{50}$'s ranging from 0.2–2.02 µg/ml (**Table 27**). Collectively, if we compare the obtained data with those of doxorubicin, it should be mentioned that tamarixellagic acid and tamgermanetin showed promising cytotoxic profiles with potent $IC_{50}$'s and R-values against all the cell lines tested herein.

Table (27): Cytotoxicity parameters of the crude extract, column fractions and isolated compounds against different solid tumor cell lines

| Fraction # | Identified Compounds | PC-3 IC$_{50}$ (µg/ml) | PC-3 R-Fr. (%) | Huh-7 IC$_{50}$ (µg/ml) | Huh-7 R-Fr. (%) | MCF-7 IC$_{50}$ (µg/ml) | MCF-7 R-Fr. (%) |
|---|---|---|---|---|---|---|---|
| Aq.alco Ext | | 6.5 | 0.0 | 2.85 | 0.55 | 0.2 | 8.4 |
| Fr. I | 3-Methoxygallic 5-OSO$_3$Na (1) | 6.2 | N/A | 11.5 | 18.2 | 2.02 | 0.0 |
| Fr. II | Kaempferide 3,7-disodium sulphate (2) | 1.5 | 6.5 | 0.84 | 0.0 | 1.2 | 0.0 |
| Fr. III | kaempferide 3-OSO$_3$Na (3), Tamarexitin 3-OSO$_3$Na (4) | 2.7 | 5.7 | 1.8 | 0.0 | 0.2 | 13.5 |
| Fr. IV | Gallic acid (5), 3-Methoxygallic acid (6) | 1.4 | 8.1 | **0.03** | 3.7 | **0.13** | 0.0 |
| Fr. V | 2,3-di-O- Galloyl-(α/β)-glucose (7) | 0.3 | 7.1 | 0.33 | 6.1 | 1.1 | 0.0 |
| Fr. VI | Quercetin 3-O-β-glucuronide (8), kaempferol 3-O-β-glucuronide (9)Tamarixetin 3-O-β-glucuronide (10) | 0.22 | 1.4 | 0.22 | 8.0 | 0.25 | 0.0 |
| Fr. VII | 1,3-di-O-Galloyl-β-glucose (11), 2,4-di-O-(α/β) Galloyl glucopyranose (12) | 0.61 | 6.7 | 0.75 | 0.0 | 0.56 | 0.0 |
| Fr. VIII | 2,6-di-O- Galloyl-(α/β)-glucose (13) | 0.4 | 0.3 | 0.13 | 10.2 | **0.15** | 0.0 |
| Fr. IX | Tamarixellagic acid (14) | **0.13** | 0.0 | **0.03** | 5.9 | **0.16** | 0.0 |
| Fr. X | kaempferol 3-O-α-rhamnopyranoside(15), Quercetin 3-O-α-rhamnopyranoside (16) | 1.3 | 2.4 | 0.9 | 4.7 | 1.9 | 0.5 |
| Fr. XI | Kaempferide (17), Tamarixetin (18), Quercetin (19) | 2.61 | 0.0 | 0.65 | 0.0 | 0.33 | 5.7 |
| Fr. XII | Tamgermanitin (20) | 0.65 | 5.1 | 0.3 | 4.1 | 1.02 | 0.0 |
| Positive control | Doxorubicin | 0.63 | 5.4 | 1.5 | 0.0 | 0.13 | 0.0 |

## 5.2. Assessment of cell cycle distribution

DNA flow-cytometry was used to assess the effect of tamarixellagic acid and tamgermanetin on the cell cycle distribution of Huh-7 and MCF-7 cell lines after treatment for 24 h. In Huh-7, tamarixellagic acid and tamgermanetin significantly decreased the non-proliferating cell fraction (G0/G1-phase) from 65% (**Fig. 64A**) to 57% (**Fig. 64B**) and 48% (**Fig. 64C**), respectively. Treatment with tamarixellagic acid induced minimal compensatory increase in S-phase while tamgermanetin showed mild increase in G2/M-phase and strong increase in the pre-G apoptotic fraction (**Fig. 64D**). With respect to MCF-7 cell line, both tamarixellagic acid (**Fig. 65B**) and tamgermanetin (**Fig. 65C**) significantly increased the pre-G apoptotic fraction compared with control (**Fig. 65A**) from 5.3–10.5% and 8.8%, respectively. Tamarixellagic acid significantly decreased the S-phase with recorded increase in response to treatment with tamgermanetin. On the other hand, tamarixellagic acid increased G2/M fraction (10.6%) while tamgermanetin depleted the mitotic cells to 2.1% compared with control cells (7.8%).

**Figure (64):** Effect of tamarixellagic acid and tamgermanitin on the cell cycle distribution of Huh-7 liver cancer cell line

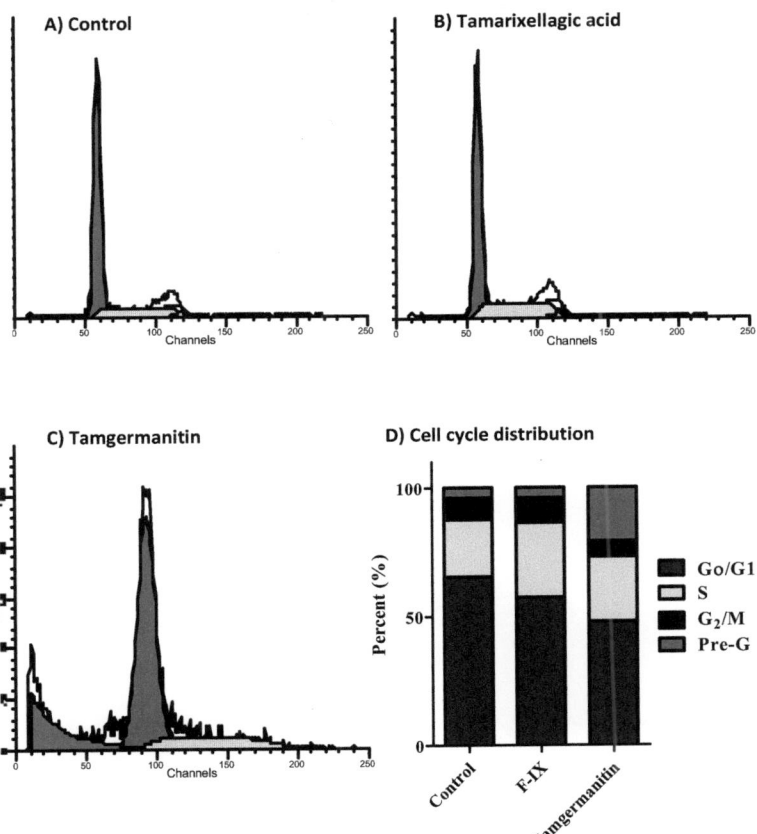

**Figure (64):** Effect of major constituent of F-IX and Tamgermanitin on the cell cycle distribution of Huh-7 cells. Cells were exposed to tamarixellagic acid (B) and tamgermanitin (C) for 24 h and compared to control cells (A). Cell cycle distribution was determined using DNA cytometry analysis and different cell phases were plotted (D) as percent of total events (n=3).

**Figure (65):** Effect of tamarixellagic acid and tamgermanitin on the cell cycle distribution of MCF-7 breast cancer cell line

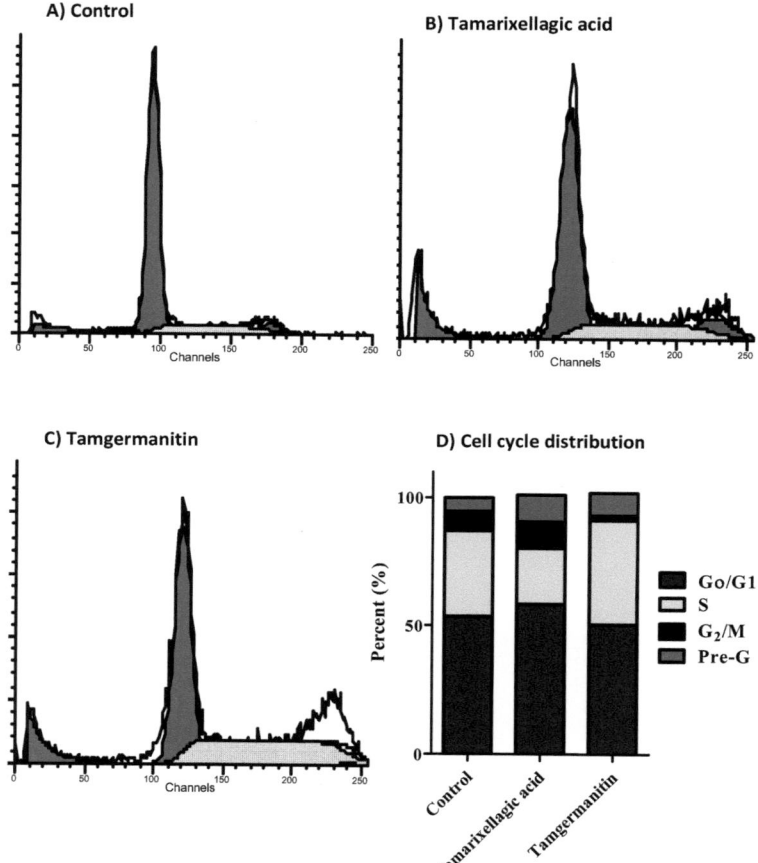

**Figure (65):** Effect of major constituent of tamarixellagic acid and tamgermanitin on the cell cycle distribution of MCF-7 cells. Cells were exposed to tamarixellagic acid (B) and tamgermanitin (C) for 24 h and compared to control cells (A). Cell cycle distribution was determined using DNA cytometry analysis and different cell phases were plotted (D) as percent of total events (n=3).

## 5.3. Assessment of PARP and caspase-3 enzyme activity.

PARP is a family of proteins involved in a number of cellular processes involving mainly DNA repair and programmed cell death and hence negatively influences apoptosis pathway after cytotoxic effects. Exposure of cell-free PARP enzyme to the pre-determined $IC_{50}$'s of tamarixellagic acid and tamgermanetin abolished the enzyme activity by 63.4 and 67.9%, respectively. The enzyme inhibition was validated by incubating the enzyme with the $IC_{50}$ of positive control PARP inhibitor (3-amino benzamide-3AB), which inhibited the enzyme by 52.1% (**Fig. 66A**). In addition to sensitizing effect of tamarixellagic acid and tamgermanetin to DNA damage, the effect on the activity of caspase-3 was assessed in Huh-7 cell line. Tamarixellagic acid and tamgermanetin increased the activity of caspase-3 activity by 154.5 and 175% respectively (**Fig. 66B**). Accordingly, tamarixellagic acid and tamgermanetin per se induce tumor cells to proceed via apoptotic pathway in addition to sensitizing tumor cells to DNA damaging agents.

**Figure (66): Effect of tamarixellagic acid and tamgermanitin on PARP and caspase-3 enzyme activity**

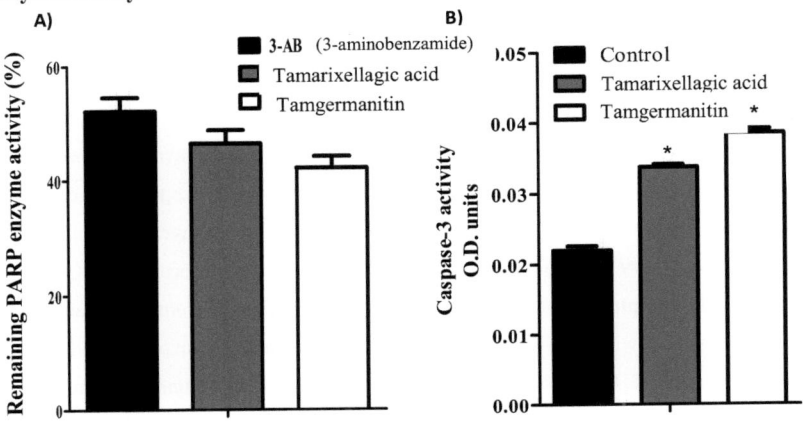

**Figure (66):** Effect of major constituent of tamarixellagic acid and tamgermanitin on PARP (A) and caspase-3 (B) enzyme activity was assessed in cell free system and in Huh-7 cell, respectively. Data are presented as mean ± SEM; (n=3).

## CONCLUSION AND RECOMMENDATION:

We present herein, a unique natural phenolic amide, $N$-isoferuloyltyramine (tamgermanitin) together with the hitherto unknown polyphenolics, 2,4-di-$O$-galloyl-($\alpha/\beta$)-glucopyranose, kaempferide 3,7-disulphate and tamarixetin 3-$O$-$\beta$-glucuronide. In addition to, 16 known phenolics have been isolated from the leaf aqueous ethanol extract of the false tamarisk, $M.$ $germanica$ with promising cytotoxic effect against three different types of solid tumors, namely, breast, prostate and liver cancers. The promising cytotoxicity of the crude extract of $M.$ $germanica$ mandated further fractionation whereby, column fractions VI and IX have shown the most promising cytotoxic profile in terms of $IC_{50}$ and R-fraction. Three flavonol glucuronoids, quercetin 3-$O$-$\beta$-glucuronide, kaempferol 3-$O$-$\beta$-glucuronide and tamarixetin 3-$O$-$\beta$-glucuronide, have been identified as the major constituents of VI. This finding might explain the superior cytotoxicity of that column fraction. Glucuronides of flavonoids are able to induce apoptosis in tested human leukaemic cells. These compounds have been reported to penetrate through cytoplasm to the nucleus of the cultured cells, and give intensive apoptotic responses in a concentration and time of incubation-related manner (Smolarz et al., 2008 ).

It is generally accepted that flavonoids prevent, delay, or help cure cancer. Thus, several reviews associating flavonoids from beverages (such as tea), fruits, vegetables, and herbals with reducing activity on cancer risk can be found (Arts, 2008; Kale et al., 2008; Le Marchand, 2002). Flavonoids can combat cancer in different, but not always clear ways. Flavonoids can prevent DNA mutations that occur in critical genes, such as oncogenes or tumor-suppressing genes, thus preventing cancer initiation or progression (Nijveldt et al., 2001). An inverse correlation has been found between dietary flavonoid intake and subsequent lung cancer occurrence (Kale et al., 2008). Quercetin (wide spread in plants, including $M germanica$) intake from onions and apples was inversely associated with the risk of having lung cancer in a study involving 9,959 Finish men and women aged 15–99, with onions being effective particularly against squamous-cell carcinoma (Le Marchand et al., 2000). It has been reported that kampferol induces apoptosis in MCF-7 cells at a concentration of 50 µM (Kang et al., 2009). This was accompanied by cleavage of PARP, as well as, the activation of caspases-7 and 9. When the cells were exposed to kaempferol, cell cycle arrest occurred at G2/M phase (Choi and Ahn, 2008). In addition flavonoids induce cell cycle arrest in prostate cancer (Haddad *et al.*, 2006).

The remarkable activity of tamarixellagic acid IX could be attributed to the typical ellagitannin monomer. More interesting is the distinguished activity determined for the unique acidamide, *N*-isoferuloyltyramine, tamgermanitin. To further substantiate the observed cytotoxicity, the potential effects of tamarixellagic acid and tamgermanitin against PARP enzyme activity were examined. Both compounds strongly inhibited the PARP enzyme activity. Distinguished role of PARP enzyme in DNA-repair and escape apoptosis has been highlighted and inhibitors of PARP enzyme sensitized several tumor types to the effect of anticancer drugs (Rios and Puhalla, 2011; Skehan *et al.*, 1990; Zhang *et al.*, 2011). Inhibition of PARP enzyme activity by tamarixellagic acid and tamgermanitin might at least partly sensitize tumor cells to death signal. This assumption is supported by the low R-fraction in all tested cell lines treated with tamarixellagic acid and tamgermanitin. Besides, tamarixellagic acid and tamgermanitin per se induced death signal as evidenced by the significant increase in the pre-G apoptotic cell fraction and the elevated caspase-3 activity in Huh-7 cell line. It is noteworthy that both materials increased the accumulation of cells at G2/M phase. This suggests that tamgermanitin-induced apoptosis might involve interaction with microtubules. This suggestion gains support by the recorded ability of amide phenolic compounds like capsaicin (Brown *et al.*, 2010; Kim *et al.*, 2010; Lee *et al.*, 2008; Lu *et al.*, 2010) and phenolic compounds like the resveratrol derivative, 2, 3'', 4, 4'', 5''-pentamethoxy-*trans*-stilbene (Belleri *et al.*, 2005; Ganapathy *et al.*, 2010) to interfere with microtubule function.

Ellagitannnins are reported to inhibit the growth of the human carcinoma cell lines KB, HeLa, DU-145, Hep 3B, and the leukemia cell line HL-60, and with little actions against normal cell line (WISH) (Wang *et al.*, 1999). Phytochemical and biological studies on ellagitannins revealed strong antitumor activity against Sarcoma-180 tumors in mice. This was exhibited by some ellagitannin oligomers including agrimoniin, oenothein B, and woodfordin C. On the other hand, some poylphenolic exhibited moderate selective cytotoxicity in *in vitro* assays using the PRMI-1951 melanoma cells (Miyamoto *et al.*, 1993; Yang *et al.*, 2000b). Hydrolyzable tannins induced S-phase arrest in both cell lines breast cancer (BCa) and prostate cancer (PCa) through inhibiting DNA replicative synthesis and G1 arrest, in addition to inducing cell death at higher levels of exposure. Hydrolzyable tannins through intraperitoneal (i.p.) injection exert a strong *in vivo* growth suppression of human PCa xenograft models in athymic nude mice. Higher levels of hydrolyzable tannins induced more caspase mediated apoptosis in MCF-7. Cell cycle arrests were achieved without an induction of cyclin-dependent kinase (CDK) inhibitory proteins P21Cip1 and P27Kip1. Penta-$O$-galloyl-$\beta$-D-glucose (PGG) treatment led to decreased cyclin D1 in both cell lines and over-expressing cyclin D1 attenuated G1 arrest and hastened S arrest. In serum-starvation synchronized MCF-7 cells, down regulation of cyclin D1 was associated with de-phosphorylation of retinoblastoma (Rb) protein by PGG shortly before G1-S transition. *In vivo,* oral administration of PGG led to a greater than 60% inhibition of MDA-MB231 xenograft growth without adverse effect on host body weight (Chai *et al.*, 2010). The potential cytotoxic effect of hydrolysable tannins of fractions V (2,3-di-$O$- galloyl-($\alpha/\beta$)-glucose, VII (1,3-di-$O$-galloyl-$\beta$-glucose, 2,4-di-$O$-($\alpha/\beta$) galloyl glucopyranose) and VIII (2,6-di-$O$- galloyl-($\alpha/\beta$)-glucose) were supported by (Chai *et al.*, 2011; Gali *et al.*, 1992).

Gallic and ellagic acids exhibits potent cytotoxicity against carcinoma cell lines and lower cytotoxicity to normal cells (Ito *et al.*, 2000; Sakagami *et al.*, 2000; Yang *et al.*, 2000a; Zunino and Capranico, 1997), this support the cytotoxic activity of fractions I and IV.

Nothing could be traced in literature regarding the cytotoxic activity of the class of sulphated flavonoids, however it is reported that flavonoids are extensively metabolized upon absorption (mostly phase II). It has been shown that flavonoid sulphates and glucuronides may at least in part be responsible for the beneficial effects of the oral intake of flavonoids. It was found that physiological levels of quercetin-3'-$O$-sulphate and quercetin-3-$O$-glucuronide (1 µM), the main circulating metabolites after consumption of quercetin-$O$-glucoside-rich diets by humans. Interestingly, only quercetin-3'-$O$-sulphate and quercetin itself were found to inhibit receptor-mediated contractions of the porcine isolated coronary artery by an endothelium-independent action, whereas quercetin-3-$O$glucuronide was inactive. Such results add to our further understanding of the complexity of the biological activities exerted by flavonoids and their metabolites as a more plausible explanation in comparison to the mere simple direct anti-oxidant activity (Ferreira *et al.*, 2010).

Recommendations:

The current study highlights a potent cytotoxic activity of the crude extract and the promising isolated compounds; tamarixellagic acid and tamgermanitin. The obtained results suggest further in-vitro investigations on the effects of these compounds on a panel of human tumor and normal cell lines. Promising activities are suggested to be further assessed in suitable animal models to define mechanism of action, effective dose levels as well as general toxicity as well as specific toxicity such as organ toxicity, mutagenicity, carcinogenicity and teratogenicity. Finally, human clinical trials will be proposed to compound(s) with acceptable profile to assess effectiveness, bioavailability, adverse effects and potential toxicity.

Zusammenfassung der Dissertation

zum Thema: „ CHEMISTRY AND BIOLOGY OF PHENOLICS ISOLATED FROM *Myricaria germanica* (L.) Desv. (Tamaricaceae) "

vorgelegt von
Noha Swilam

# SUMMARY

In accordance with the recent worldwide interest in plant phenolics, which emerges from their broad range of biological activities, particular emphasis has been focused, in the present thesis, on the constitutive phenolics of the extract of *Myricaria germanica* (L.) Desv. (Tamaricaceae).

During the current thesis twenty phenolics (**1 – 20**) were isolated and identified from the aqueous/ethanol extract of the whole *Myricaria germanica* plant. The isolates include four hitherto unknown natural phenolics (**2, 10, 12** and **20**). Also, the cytotoxic activities of *M. germanica* extract, column fractions, and one new natural isolate against three different solid tumor cell lines, namely, breast cancer (MCF-7), prostate (PC-3), and liver (Huh-7) cancer cell using SRB viability assay have been investigated and first insights into mode of action have been obtained.

**Phytochemical investigation**

The phytochemical study of *Myricaria germanica* included successive column chromatographic investigation of the aqueous/alcohol aerial parts extract, separation of individual phenolics, repeated purification of these individuals and establishment of their homogeneity by paper chromatography. For structure elucidation, the required structural information was obtained through chromatographic analysis, application of chemical degradation methods and conventional spectroscopic techniques of analysis as well. Besides, mass spectrometric and nuclear magnetic resonance spectroscopic analytical techniques were extensively applied in this thesis, either to unravel the chemical structure of the isolated new natural phenolics, to clarify the full structure of some of the known phenolics and to get no previously reported spectral data for some others. As a result of this intensive study, twenty phenolic constituents were individually isolated and identified, ten of which have not been previously identified in *Myricaria germanica*; among them four compounds were found to be new natural products. Isolate **20** was of special interest due to its unique structure. The new compounds were identified to be:

Compound **2**, Kaempferide 3, 7- sodium disulphate

Compound **10**, Tamarixetin 3-*O*-β-glucupyranuronoide

Compound **12**, 2, 4- di-*O*-Galloyl-(α/β)-$^4C_1$-glucopyranose

Compound **20**, *N-trans*-3-hydroxy 4-methoxy cinnamoyltyramine, a unique isoferuloyl derivative, for which we gave the name Tamgermanetin.

# SUMMARY

[Chemical structure diagram showing a compound with a hydroxyphenyl-ethylamine linked via an amide to a cinnamoyl group bearing OMe and OH substituents; positions numbered 1–9, 1'–8', 2'–6'.]

In addition, the known compounds, 3-Methoxy gallic acid 5-sodium sulphate (**1**), Kaempferide 3-sodium sulphate (**3**), Tamarexitin 3-sodium sulphate (**4**), Gallic acid (**5**), 3-Methoxygallic acid (**6**), 2,3-di-*O*-Galloyl-(α/β)-$^4C_1$-glucopyranose (**7**), Quercetin 3-*O*-β-$^4C_1$-glucuronide (**8**), Kaempferol 3-*O*-β-$^4C_1$-glucuronide (**9**), 1,3-di-*O*-Galloyl-β-glucose (**11**), 2,6-di-*O*-Galloyl-(α/β)-$^4C_1$-glucopyranose (**13**), Tamarixellagic acid (**14**), Kaempferol 3-*O*-α-rhamnopyranoside (**15**), Quercetin 3-*O*-α-rhamnopytanoside (**16**), Kaempferol (**17**), Kaempferide (**17***), Tamarixetin (**18**) and Quercetin (**19**) were also isolated and identified by applying the conventional and spectral methods of analysis.

## Biological investigation of *Myricaria germanica* aerial parts extract, column fractions and isolated compounds

### Cytotoxicity assessment:

SRB-U assay was used to assess the cytotoxicity of the crude extract and its fractions against three different tumor cell lines over range 0.01–100 µg/ml. Doxorubicin was used as a positive control. The crude extract per se showed considerable potency against PC-3, Huh-7 and MCF-7 cell lines with IC50 values of 6.5, 2.85 and 0.2 µg/ml, respectively. MCF-7 cell line showed relatively high resistance fraction after treatment with the crude extract with R-fraction of 8.4% while there were negligible R-values for PC-3 and Huh-7 cells (0 and 0.55%, respectively). Collectively, if we compare the obtained data with those of doxorubicin, it should be mentioned that tamarixellagic acid and tamgermanetin showed promising cytotoxic profiles with potent $IC_{50}$'s and R-values against all the cell lines tested herein.

# SUMMARY

**Assessment of cell cycle distribution:**

DNA flow-cytometry was used to assess the effect of tamarixellagic acid and tamgermanetin on the cell cycle distribution of Huh-7 and MCF-7 cell lines after treatment for 24 h. In Huh-7, tamarixellagic acid and tamgermanetin significantly decreased the non-proliferating cell fraction (G0/G1-phase) from 65% to 57% and 48% respectively. Both tamarixellagic acid and tamgermanetin significantly increased the pre-G apoptotic fraction compared with control from 5.3–10.5% and 8.8%, respectively.

**Assessment of PARP and caspase-3 enzyme activity:**

Exposure of cell-free PARP enzyme to the pre-determined $IC_{50}$'s of tamarixellagic acid and tamgermanetin abolished the enzyme activity by 63.4 and 67.9%, respectively. In addition to sensitizing effect of tamarixellagic acid and tamgermanetin to DNA damage, the effect on the activity of caspase-3 was assessed in Huh-7 cell line. Tamarixellagic acid and tamgermanetin increased the caspase-3 activity by 154.5 and 175% respectively. Accordingly, tamarixellagic acid and tamgermanetin per se induce tumor cells to proceed via apoptotic pathway in addition to sensitizing tumor cells to DNA damaging agents

## ZUSAMMENFASSUNG

Phenolische Pflanzeninhaltsstoffe zeichnen sich durch ein breites Spektrum an biologischen Aktivitäten aus und gewinnen aufgrund dessen großes Interesse für die Prävention und Behandlung verschiedener Erkrankungen. Besondere Aufmerksamkeit verdienen Verbindungen aus ethnomedizinisch verwendeten Pflanzen, die bisher nicht oder nur unzureichend phytochemisch untersucht worden sind. Zu diesen Pflanzen gehört *Myricaria germanica* (L.) Desv.. In der vorliegenden Arbeit werden die konstitutiven Phenole des Extraktes von *Myricaria germanica* (L.) Desv. (Tamaricaceae) chemisch analysiert und auf biologische Aktivität geprüft. Aus dem wässrig-ethanolischen Extrakt der gesamten oberirdischen Pflanze wurden zwanzig Phenole (**1 - 20**) isoliert und identifiziert. Dabei wurden vier bisher unbekannte natürliche Phenole (**2, 10, 12** und **20**) aufgefunden. Die biologischen Untersuchungen konzentrierten sich auf die zytotoxischen Aktivitäten des Extraktes, der Fraktionen und einiger isolierter Verbindungen gegen drei verschiedene Tumor-Zelllinien, nämlich Brustkrebs (MCF-7), Prostatakrebs (PC-3) und Leber (Huh-7) Krebszellen, die mit Hilfe des SRB Assays untersucht wurden. Darüber hinaus wurden Informationen zum Wirkungsmechanismus gewonnen.

**Phytochemische Untersuchung**

Die Isolierung der phenolischen Inhaltsstoffe von *Myricaria germanica* erfolgte durch aufeinander folgende säulenchromatographische Trennungen des wässrig/alkoholischen Extrakts der oberirdischen Teile der Pflanze, die Abtrennung einzelner Phenole, die wiederholte Reinigung dieser Substanzen und die Ermittlung ihrer Reinheit durch chromatographische Verfahren. Für die Strukturaufklärung wurden die erforderlichen Informationen durch chromatographische Analyse, Anwendung von chemischen Abbauverfahren und konventionelle spektroskopische Techniken erhalten. Außerdem wurde ausführliche massenspektrometrische und NMR- spektroskopische Analyseverfahren angewendet, um entweder die chemische Struktur der isolierten neuen natürlichen Phenole zu klären oder um die volle Struktur der bekannten Phenole zu analysieren. Als Ergebnis der intensiven Studie wurden zwanzig phenolische Bestandteile isoliert und identifiziert. Zehn von ihnen wurden zum ersten Mal in *Myricaria germanica* nachgewiesen. Bei vier Verbindungen handelt es sich um neue, bisher nicht beschriebene Naturstoffe.

ZUSAMMENFASSUNG

Aufgrund seiner einzigartigen Struktur war Isolat 20 von besonderem Interesse. Die neuen Verbindungen wurden identifiziert als:

Verbindung **2**, Kaempferid 3, 7- natriumdisulfat

Verbindung **10**, Tamarixetin 3-*O*-β-glucopyranuronid

Verbindung **12,** 2, 4-di-*O*-Galloyl-(α / β)-$^4C_1$-glucopyranose, ein neuer hydrolysierbarer Gerbstoff

ZUSAMMENFASSUNG

Verbindung **20**, N-*trans*-3-Hydroxy-4-methoxy cinnamoyltyramine, wofür wir den Namen Tamgermanetin vorschlagen.

Darüber hinaus wurden die bekannten Verbindungen 3-Methoxy-gallussäure-5-natriumsulfat (**1**), Kaempferid-3-natriumsulfat (**3**), Tamarexitin 3-natriumsulfat (**4**), Gallussäure (**5**), 3-Methoxy-gallussäure (**6**), 2,3-di-*O*-Galloyl-(α / β)-$^4C_1$-glucopyranose (**7**), Quercetin 3-*O*-3 - $^4C_1$-glucuronid (**8**), Kaempferol 3 - *O*-β - $^4C_1$-glucuronid (**9**), 1, 3-di-*O*-Galloyl-β-glucose (**11**), 2, 6-di-*O*-Galloyl-(α / β)-$^4C_1$-glucopyranose (**13**), Tamarixellagicssäure (**14**), Kaempferol 3-*O*-α-rhamnopyranoside (**15**), Quercetin-3-*O*-α-rhamnopytanoside (**16**), Kaempferol (**17**), Kaempferid (**17\***), Tamarixetin (**18**) und Quercetin (**19**) isoliert und durch Anwendung strukturanalytischer Analysemethoden identifiziert.

**Biologische Untersuchung des Extraktes der oberirdischen Teile von Myricaria germanica, der Säulenfraktionen und der isolierten Verbindungen**

**Zytotoxizität:**

Die Zytotoxizität der Proben im Konzentrationsbereich von 0,01 bis 100 µg/ml wurde mithilfe des SRB-U-Test gegen 3 Tumorzelllinien (PC-3, Huh-7 und MCF-7–Zellen) untersucht. Doxorubicin wurde als positive Kontrolle verwendet. Der Rohextrakt zeigte mit $IC_{50}$ -Werten von 6,5 , 2,85 und 0,2 µg / ml gegen die drei Zelllinien beträchtliche Zytotoxizität. Die MCF-7–Zellen wiesen nach der Behandlung mit dem Rohextrakt einen relativ hohen Anteil der R- Fraktion von 8,4 % auf, während es unerhebliche R- Werte für die PC-3 und Huh-7-Zellen (0 bzw. 0,55 %) gab. Im Vergleich mit Doxorubicin zeigen Tamarixellagsäure und Tamgermanetin vielversprechende zytotoxische Profile mit potenten

IC$_{50}$ und R- Werten gegen alle getesteten Zelllinien.

**Zellzyklus:**

Die Durchflusszytometrie wurde verwendet, um die Wirkung von Tamarixellagsäure und Tamgermanetin auf die Zellzyklus-Verteilung von Huh-7 und MCF-7-Zelllinien nach Behandlung über 24 h zu bewerten. In Huh-7-Zellen verringern Tamarixellagsäure und Tamgermanetin signifikant den Anteil der nicht-proliferierenden Zellfraktion (G0/G1-Phase) von 65% auf 57% bzw. 48%. Sowohl Tamarixellagsäure als auch Tamgermanetin erhöhen signifikant den Anteil pre-G apoptotischer Zellen verglichen mit der Kontrollgruppe von 5,3 auf 10,5 % und beziehungsweise 8,8 %.

**PARPundCaspase-3-Enzymaktivität:**

Tamarixellagsäure und Tamgermanetin hemmten in der jeweiligen IC$_{50}$-Konzentration in einem zellfreien System die Enzymaktivität von PARP um 63,4 bzw. 67,9 %. Die Aktivität von Caspase-3 in der Huh-7-Zelllinie wurde durch Tamarixellagsäure und Tamgermanetin auf 154,5 bzw. 175 % erhöht. Daraus lässt sich auf eine Apoptoseinduzierende Wirkung der Verbindungen schließen.

Hiermit erkläre ich, dass diese Arbeit bisher von mir weder an der Mathematisch-Naturwissenschaftlichen Fakultät der Ernst-Moritz-Arndt-Universität Greifswald noch einer anderen wissenschaftlichen Einrichtung zum Zwecke der Promotion eingereicht wurde.

Ferner erkläre ich, dass ich diese Arbeit selbständig verfasst und keine anderen als die darin angegebenen Hilfsmittel und Hilfen benutzt und keine Textabschnitte eines Dritten ohne Kennzeichnung übernommen habe.

Noha Swilam

# REFERENCES

Ahemad AF, Memon MU, Yoshida T and Okuda T (1994) Part VI :Four trimeric tannins from *Reaumuria hirtella* and *Tamarix pakistanica*. *Chem Pharm Bull* **42**:254-264.

Ahmad M, Ahmad W, Khan S, Zeeshan M, Obaidullah, Nisar M and Shaheen F (2008) New antibacterial pentacyclic triterpenes from *Myricaria elegans* Royle. (tamariscineae). *Journal of enzyme inhibition and medicinal chemistry* **23**:1023-1027.

Ai C, Wen Q and Sang J (2000) A Tibetan medicated bath lotion for treating rheumatic arthritis, rheumatoid arthritis, chronic pain of low back and legs, and dermatoses. *Faming Zhuanli Shenqing*.

Akagawa M and Suyama K (2001) Amine oxidase-like activity of polyphenols: Mechanism and properties. *Eur J Biochem* **268**:1953.

Anne MF (2000) Oligomeric proanthocyanidin complexes: history, structure, and phytopharmaceutical applications. *Altern Med Rev* **5**:144.

Arts ICW (2008) A review of the epidemiological evidence on tea, flavonoids, and lung cancer. *J Nutr*:1561–1566.

Asanaka M, Kurimura T, Kushiura R, Okuda T, Mori M and Yokoi H (1988) Tannins as candidates for anti-HIV drug. *Int J Immunopharmaco* **10**:35.

Baily LH (1950) *The Standard Cyclopedia of Horticulture*, MacMillan & Co, New York.

Baima Z, Zhang Y, Zhang G, Chen L and Zhang Q (2011) Application of a Tibetan medicine composition in preparation of drugs for treating central neurogenic pains. *Faming Zhuanli Shenqing*.

Barron D, Varin L, Ibrahim R and J. H (1988a) Sulphated flavonoids-an update. *Phytochemistry* **27**:2375-2395.

BD FACSVerse System User's Guide. 23-11463-00 Rev. 01

Belleri M, Ribatti D, Nicoli S, Cotelli F, Forti L, Vannini V, Stivala L and Presta M (2005) Antiangiogenic and vascular-targeting activity of the microtubule-destabilizing *trans*-resveratrol derivative 3,5,4'-trimethoxystilbene. *Mol Pharmacol* **67**:1451-1459.

Bohle K.: Distribution and abundance of rare plant communities in Vorarlberg. Part 2 Dwarf cattail reeds (Equiseto-Typhetum minimae) and Myrtengebüsche (Salici-Myricarietum). Thesis, University of Innsbruck 1987

Bouchet N, Barrier L and Fauconneau B (1998) Radical scavenging activity and antioxidant properties of tannins from *Guiera senegalensis* (Combretaceae)". *Phytothr Res* **12**:159-162.

Boulos L (1983) *Medicinal Plants of North Africa*, Michiga.

Boulos L (1999) Flora of Egypt, Vol.1,Al-Hadara Publishing, Cairo,Egypt.

Brown DM, Kelly GE and Husband AJ (2005) Flavonoid compounds in maintenance of prostate health and prevention and treatment of cancer. *Mol Biotechnol* **30**:253-270.

Brown K, Witte T, Hardman W, Luo H and Chen Y (2010) Capsaicin displays anti-proliferative activity against human small cell lung cancer in cell culture and Nude Mice models via the E2F Pathway. *PLoS ONE* **5**:10243.

Brown MD (1999) Green Tea (*Camellia Sinensis*) extract and its possible role in the prevention of cancer. *Altern Med Rev* **4**:360.

Brynin R (2002) Soy and its isoflavones: A Review of their effects on bone density. *Altern Med Rev* **7**:317.

Chai Y, Lee H, Shaik A, Nkhati K, Xing C, Zhang J, Jeong S, Kim S and Lü J (2011) Penta-O-galloyl-b-D-glucose induces G1 arrest and DNA replicative S-phase arrest independently of P21 cyclin-dependent kinase inhibitor 1A, P27 cyclin-dependent kinase inhibitor 1B and P53 in human breast cancer cells and is orally active against triple-negative xenograft growth. *Breast Cancer Research* **12**.

Choi EJ and Ahn WS (2008) Kaempferol induced the apoptosis via cell cycle arrest in human breast cancer MDA-MB-453 cells. *Nutr Res Pract* **2**:322–325.

Chopra RN, Nayar SL and Chopra IC (1956) *Glossary of Indian Medicinal Plants*, New Delhi.

Choueiri TK, Mekhail T, Hutson TE, Ganapathi R, Kelly.G.E. and Bukowski RM (2006) Phase I trial of phenoxodiol delivered by continuous intravenous infusion in patients with solid cancer. *Annals of Oncology* **17**:860-865.

Christiane K and Johannes K (2012) Clonal re-introduction of endangered plant species: the case of German False Tamarisk in pre-alpine rivers. *Environmental management* **50**:217-225.

Chumbalov TK, Bikbulatova TN and Il'yasova MI (1974) Polyphenols of *Myricaria alopecuroides*. *Khimiya Prirodnykh Soedinenii* **3**.

Chumbalov TK, Bikbulatova TN and Il'yasova MI (1976) Polyphenols from *Myricaria alopecuroides*. III. Hydrolyzable tanning substances. *Khimiya Prirodnykh Soedinenii* **1**:131-132. Language: Russian.

Chumbalov TK, Bikbulatova TN and Il'yasova MI (1979) Polyphenols of *Myricaria*. IV. Hydrolyzed tannin. *Khimiya Prirodnykh Soedinenii* **1**:107 Language: Russian.,

Chumbalov TK, Bikbulatova TN, Il'yasova MI and Mukhamedieva RM (1975) Polyphenols of *Myricaria alopecuroides*. II. Flavonoid aglycons. *Khimiya Prirodnykh Soedinenii* **11**:282-283. Language: Russian.

Clark B and Lama D (1995) *The quintessence Tantras of Tibetan Medicine*, Snow Lion publication, New York, USA.

De Bruyn A, Auteunis M and von Beeumen J (1977a) Chemical shifts of aldohexopyranoses revisited and application to gulosylglucose. Bull soc chim Belg 86:259.

Decker JP (1961) Salt secretion by *Tamarix pentandra*. *Pall Forest Science* **7**:214-217.

Dudek-Makuch M and Matawska I (2011) Flavonoids from the flowers of *Aesculus hippocastanum*. *Acta Poloniae Pharmaceutica* - Drug Research **68**:403-408.

Duo J (2011) Processing method of Tibetan medicine iron powder and its application. *Faming Zhuanli Shenqing*.

El Ansari MA, Nawwar MAM, El Sherbeiny AEA and El-Sissi HI (1976) A sulphated kaempferol 7, 4' - dimethyl ether and a quercetin isoferulyl glucuronide from the flowers of *Tamarix aphylla*. *Phytochemistry* **15**:231-232.

El-Mousallamy AM, Hussein SA, Merfort I and Nawwar MA (2000) Unusual phenolic glycosides from *Cotoneaster orbicularis*. *Phytochemistry* **53** 6:699-704.

El-Sissi HI, Nawwar MAM and Saleh NAM (1973) Plant constituents of *Tamarix nilotica* leaves (Tamaricaceae). **29**:1064.

Fairbrain JW (1942) Pharmj 148:198.

Farnsworth NR (1954) *J Pharm Sci* 55:265-266.

Feldman KS (2005) Recent progress in ellagitannin chemistry. *Phytochemistry* **66**:1984–2000.

Ferreira J, Luthria D, Sasaki T and Heyerick A (2010) Flavonoids from *Artemisia annua* L. as antioxidants and their potential synergism with Artemisinin against Malaria and Cancer. *Molecules* **15**:3135-3170.

Frisendahl A. *Myricaria germanica* (L.) Acta DESV *Florae Sueciae*. **1**: 265-304, 1921

Fukushi K, Sakagami H, Okuda T, Hatano T, Tanuma S, Kitajima K, Inuoe Y, Inuoe S, Ishikawa S, Nonoyama M and Konno K (1989) Inhibition of herpes simplex virus infection by tannins and related compounds. *Antiviral Res* **11**:285.

Fulton CC (1932) *Amer J Pharm* 104:144.

# REFRENCES

G. Hegi (1975): *Illustrated Flora of Central Europe*. Volume 5, Part 1: Dicotyledones, Linaceae - Violaceae. Verlag Paul Parey, Berlin, Hamburg.

Gali HU, Perchellet EM, Klish DS, Johnson JM and Perchelle JP (1992) Antitumorpromoting activities of hydrolyzable tannins in mouse skin. *Carcinogenesis* **13**.

Ganapathy S, Chen Q, Singh K, Shankar S and Srivastava R (2010) Resveratrol Enhances Antitumor Activity of TRAIL in Prostate Cancer Xenografts through Activation of FOXO Transcription Factor. . *PLoS ONE* **5**:15627.

Geissman TA (1966) *The Chemistry of Flavonoid Compounds*, Pergamon Press, London.

Germano MP, D'Angelo V, Sanogo R, Catania S, Alma R, De Pasquale R and Bisignaro G (2005) Hepatoprotective and antibacterial effects of extracts from *Trichilia emetica* Vahl. (Meliaceae). *J of Ethnopharmacology* **96**:227.

Gonzales EE and Delango JN (1962) *J Pharm Sci* **51**.

Gupta RK, Al-Shafi S, Layden K and Haslam E (1982) The metabolism of gallic acid and hexahydroxydiphenic acid in plants. Part 2. Esters of (S)-hexahydroxydiphenic acid with D-glucopyranose ($^4C_1$). *J Chem Soc Perkin Trans* **I**:2525.

Haddad AQ, Venkateswaren V, Viswanathen L, Teahan SJ, Flesher NE and Klotz LH (2006) Novel antiproliferative flavonoids induce cell cycle arrest in prostate cancer. *Prostate cancer Prostatic diseases* **9**:68-76.

Haddock A, Gupta K, Al-Shafi M and Haslam E (1982a) The metabolism of gallic acid and hexahydrooxydiphenic acid in plants. Part 1. Introduction. Naturally occuring galloyl esters. *J Chem Sot Perkin Trans* **1**:2515..

Hagimasi K, Blazovics A and Feher J (2000) The *in vitro* effect of dandelions antioxidants on microsomal lipid peroxidation. *Phytothr Res* **14**:43-44.

Harborne J and Williams C eds (1975) *The Flavonoids*, Chapman & Hall, London.

Harborne JB (1973) *Phytochemical Methods*, Chapman and Hall, London.

Harborne JB (1973) *Phytochemical Methods*, Chapman and Hall, London.

Harborne JB (1982) *The Flavonoids: Advances in Research*, Chapman and Hall, London.

Harborne JB and William CA (1975) *The Flavonoids*, "T", Chapman and Hall, London.

Harvey AL (1999) Medicines from nature: are natural products still relevant to drug discovery? *Trends Pharmacol Sci* **20**:196-198.

Haslam E (1996) Natural polyphenols (vegetable tannins) as drugs: Possible modes of action. *J Nat Prod* **59**:205.

# REFRENCES

Haslam E, Lilley TH, Cai Y, Martin R and Magnolato D (1989) Traditional herbal medicines - the role of polyphenols. *Planta medica* **55**:1.

Hawkins PJ (1958) What trees to plant on the downs. *Queensland Agri J* **84**:368- 374.

He J (2009) Traditional Chinese medicinal composition for treating tinea pedis and tinea manus, and preparation method thereof. *Faming Zhuanli Shenqing*.

Hemingway RW, Gross GG and Yoshida T (1999) "Plant Polyphenols: Chemistry and Biology Plenum Press, New York.

Herriot R (1942) The athel trees, an evergreen Tamarisk. *Austral Dept Agr J* **46**: 58-59.

Hutchinson J (1967) *The Genera of Flowering Plants*, Oxford.

Imperato F (1979) Two new kaempferol 3,7-diglycosides and kaempferitrin in the fern *Asplenium trichomanes*. *Experientia* **35**:1134.

Ito H, Kobayashi E, Takamatsu Y, Li S-H, Hatano T, Sakagami H, Kusama K, Satoh K, Ugita D, Shimura S, Itoh Y and Yoshida T (2000) Polyphenols from *Eriobotrya japonica* and Their Cytotoxicity against Human Oral Tumor Cell Lines. *Chem Pharm Bull* **48**:687–693.

Jetter R (2000) Long-chain alkanediols from Myricaria germanica leaf cuticular waxes. *Phytochemistry* **55**:169-176.

Jiang Z, Hirose Y, Iwata H, Sakamoto S, Tanaka T and Kouno I (2001) Caffeoyl, Coumaroyl, Galloyl, and Hexahydroxydiphenoyl Glucoses from *Balanophora japonica*. *Chem Pharm Bull* **49**:887-892.

Jiumei P (2001) A Tibetan medicinal composition for the treatment of hepatitis, and preparation method thereof. *Faming Zhuanli Shenqing*.

Jiumei P (2006) A Chinese medicinal composition granule for medicated bath, and its preparation method. *Faming Zhuanli Shenqing*.

Jurd L (1962) *Chemistry of the Flavonoid Compounds*, Geisman, T. A. (Ed.), Pergamon Press, Oxford.

Kale A, Gawande S and Kotwal S (2008) Cancer phytotherapeutics: role for flavonoids at the cellular level. *Phytoth Res* **22**: 567–577.

Kang G-Y, Lee E-R, Kim J-H, Jung JW, Lim J, Kim SK, Cho S-G and Kim KP (2009) Downregulation of PLK-1 expression in kaempferol-induced apoptosis of MCF-7 cells. *Eur JPharmacol* **611**:17–21.

Khan S, Nisar M, Khan R, Ahmad W and Nasir F (2010) Evaluation of chemical constituents and antinociceptive properties of *Myricaria elegans* Royle. *Chemistry & biodiversity* **7**:2897-2900.

Khyade MS, Awasarkar UD, Deshmukh RR and Petkar AS (2010) Ethnobotanical reports about few important diseases from Akole Tehasil Ahmednagar District (MS) India. *ASIAN J EXP BIOL SCI* **1**:393-403.

Kim K, Choi S, Son M and KR. L (2010) Two new phenolic amides from the seeds of *Pharbitis nil*. *Chem Pharm Bull* (Tokyo) **59**:1532-1535.

King R and Calhoun L (2005) Characterization of cross-linked hydroxycinnamic acid amides isolated from potato common scab lesions. *Phytochemistry* **66**:2468-2473.

Kirbag S, Zengin F and Kursat M (2009) Antimicrobial activities of extracts of some plants. *Pak J Bot* **41**:2067-2070.

Ksouri R, Falleh H, Megdiche W, Trabelsi N, Mhamdi B, Chaieb K, Bakrouf A, Christian Magné C and Abdelly C (2009) Antioxidant and antimicrobial activities of the edible medicinal halophyte *Tamarix gallica* L. and related polyphenolic constituents. *Food and Chemical Toxicology* **47**:2083–2091.

La X, Zeng Y and Xu M (2011) Flavonoids in *Myricaria germanica* of Tibetan medicine. *Tianran Chanwu Yanjiu Yu Kaifa* **23**:596-599.

Lawrence GHM (1951) *Taxonomy of Vascular Plants*, The MacMillan Company, New York.

Le Marchand L (2002) Cancer preventive effects of flavonoids-a review. *Biomed Pharmacother* **56**:296–301.

Le Marchand L, Murphy SP, Hankin JH, Wilkens LR and Kolonel LN (2000) Intake of flavonoids and lung cancer. *J Natl Cancer Inst* **92**:154–160.

Lee H, Yang L, Xu J, Ying S, Yeung V, Huang Y and Chen Z (2005) Relative antioxidant activity of soybean isoflavones and their glycosides. *Food Chemistry* **90**:735.

Lee K, Yang M, Kim K, Kwon H, Choi S and Lee K (2008) A new phenolic amide from the Roots of *Paris verticillata*. *molecules* **13**:41-45.

Lee TI, Jenner RG, Boyer LA, Guenther MG, Levine SS, Kumar RM, Chevalier B, Johnstone SE, Cole MF and Isono K (2006) Control of developmental regulators by polycomb in human embryonic stem cells. *Cell* **15**:301-313.

Lei J (2005) Tibetan medicinal composition for treating acute and chronic sprain and contusion, rheumatism and rheumatoid diseases, and its preparation method. *Faming Zhuanli Shenqing*.

Lei J and Zhang Y (2005) A salt-containing Tibetan medicinal composition having therapeutic and health protection effects, and preparation method thereof. *Faming Zhuanli Shenqing*.

# REFRENCES

Lei J, Lamu Y and Su B (1999) Method for processing natural plant medicinal bath foam into powdered medicine. *Faming Zhuanli Shenqing*.

Lei J, Zhang Y, Chen L, Zhu J and Liu H (2008a) A medicated toothpaste containing Lamiophlomis rotata extract and having therapeutic effect on oral disease, and its preparation method. *Faming Zhuanli Shenqing*.

Lei J, Zhang Y, Zhu J, Chen L and Liu H (2008b) Medical toothpaste of gypsum rubrum and its preparation process. *Faming Zhuanli Shenqing*.

Leiber mann C and Burchard H (1890) *Chem Zentre* 61.

Li J, Zhang G, Chen L, Zhang Y and Wang Y (2011) Traditional chinese medicine composition for treating bronchial asthma. *Faming Zhuanli Shenqing*.

Li S, Chen RY and Yu DQ (2007) [Study on chemical constituents of Myricaria paniculata I]. *Zhongguo Zhong yao za zhi = Zhongguo zhongyao zazhi = China journal of Chinese materia medica* **32**:403-406.

Li S, Dai SJ, Chen RY and Yu DQ (2005) Triterpenoids from the stems of *Myricaria paniculata*. *Journal of Asian natural products research* **7**:253-257.

Li X and Liu Y (2009) Tibetan medicine aerosol for treating acute/chronic sprain, contusion, rheumatosis and rheumatoid disease. *Faming Zhuanli Shenqing*.

Li Z, Xue P, Xie H, Li X and Xie M (2010) [Chemical constituents from *Myricaria alopecuroides*]. *Zhongguo Zhong yao za zhi = Zhongguo zhongyao zazhi = China journal of Chinese materia medica* **35**:865-868.

Lu H, Chen Y, Yang J, Yang Y, Liu J, Hsu S and Chung J (2010) Antitumor activity of capsaicin on human colon cancer cells *in Vitro* and Colo 205 Tumor Xenografts *in Vivo*. *J Agric Food Chem* **58**:12999-13005.

Mabberley DI (1987) *The Plant Book*, Camb. Univ. Press, Cambridge, New York.

Mabry TJ, Markham KR and Thomas MB (1969) *The Systematic Identification of the Flavonoids*, Springer, New York.

Markham K, Ternai B, Stanley R, Geiger H and Mabry T (1978) Carbon-13 NMR studies of flavonoids-III. *Tetrahedron Letters* **34**:1389–1397.

Miyamoto K, Kishi, N, Koshiura R, Yoshida T, Hatano T and Okuda T (1987) Relationship between the structures and the antitumor activities of tannins. *Chem Pharm Bull* **35**:814.

Miyamoto K, Murayama T, Nomura M, Hatano T, Yoshida T, Furukawa T, Koshiura R and Okuda T (1993a) Antitumor activity and interleukin-1 induction by tannins. *Anticancer Res* **13**:37–42.

Miyamoto K, Nomura M, Murayama T, Furukawa T, Hatano T, Yoshida T, Koshiura R and Okuda T (1993) Antitumor activities of ellagitannins against sarcoma-180 in mice. *Biol Pharm Bull* **16**.

Miyamoto K, Nomura M, Sasakura M, Matsui E, Koshiura R, Murayama T, Furukawa T, Hatano T, Yoshida T and Okuda T (1993b) Antitumor activity of oenothein B, a unique macrocyclic ellagitannin. *Jpn J Cancer Res* **84**: 99–103.

Molisch J (1886) *Montash Chem* 7:198.

Moore GE, Mount DT and Wendt AC (1958) The growth of human tumor cells in tissue culture. *Surg Forum* **9**:572-576.

Morazzoni P and Bombvardelli E (1996) *Vaccinium myrtillus* L. *Fitoterapia* 67:3.

Mozingo HN (1987) *Shrubs of the Great Basin: A natural history*, NV:University of Nevada Press, Reno.

Mukkerjee S and Srivasttava HC (1952) Improved spray reagent for the detection of sugar. *Nature* **169**:330.

Müller N and Citizen A (1990): riverbed morphology and riparian vegetation of the Lech in the Forch Acher Wildflusslandschaft (Upper Lech Valley, Tirol) Association for the Protection of the mountains, 55. 43-74, Munich

Nadkarni AK (1976) *Indian Materia Medica*, Bombay.

Nawwar M and Buddrus J (1981) A gossypetin glucuronide sulphate from the leaves of *Malva sylvestris*. *Phytochemistry* **20**:2446.

Nawwar M and Hussein S (1994) Gall polyphenolics of *Tamarix aphylla*. *Phytochemistry* **36**:1035-1037.

Nawwar M, Buddrus J and Bauer H (1982) Dimeric phenolic constituents from the roots of **Tamarix nilotica**. *Phytochemistry* **21**:1755-1758.

Nawwar M, El-Ansary M, El Sherbieny A and El-Sissi H (1976) Sulphated kaempferol 7,4'-dimethyl ether and a quercetin isoferulyl glucuronoide from the flowers of *Tamarix aphylla*. *Phytochemistry* **15**: 231-232.

Nawwar M, Hussein S, Buddrus J and Linscheid M (1994a) Tamarixellagic acid, an ellagitannin from the galls of *Tamarix aphylla*. *Phytochemistry* **35**:1349-1354.

Nawwar M, Souleman A, Buddrus J, Bauer H and Linscheid M (1984) Polyphenolic constituents of the flowers of *Tamarix nilotica* : The structure of nilocitin, a new digalloylglucoside. *Tetrahedron Letters* **23**:2347-2349

Nawwar MAM, Hussein SAM and Merfort I (1994b) NMR Specteral analysis of polyphenols from *Punica granatum*. *Phytochemistry* **30**:793-798.

Nawwar MAM, Ishak MS, Michael HN and Buddrus J (1984b) Leaf flavonoids of *Ziziphus spina-christi*. *Phytochemistry* **23**:2110-2111.

Nawwar MAM, Souleman AMA, Buddrus J and Linscheid M (1984d) Flavonoids of the flowers of *Tamarix nilotica*. *Phytochemistry* **23**:2347- 2349.

Neich AC (1960) *Biosynthetic Pathways of Aromatic Compounds*. Annual Rev Pl Physiol.

Nijveldt RJ, van Nood E, van Hoorn DEC, Boelens PG, van Norren K and van Leeuwen PAM (2001) Flavonoids: a review of probable mechanisms of action and potential applications. *Am J Clin Nutr* 74:418–425.

Nitta T, Arai T, Takamatsu H, Iinuma M, Tanaka, T. I, T., Asai F, Ibrahim I, Nakanishi T and Watabe K (2002) Antibacterial activity of extracts prepared from tropical and subtropical plants on Methicillin-Resistant *Staphylococcus aureus*. *J Health Sci* **48**:273.

Nonaka G, Sakai R and Nishioka I (1984) Hydrolyzable tannins and proanthocyanidins from green tea. *Phytochemistry* **23**:1753 - 1755

Okuda T, Yoshida T and Hatano T (1989) New Methods of Analyzing Tannin. *J Nat Prod* 52:1–31.

Okuda T, Yoshida T and Hatano T (1990) Oligomeric hydrolysable tannins a new class of plant polyphenols. *Heterocycles* **30**:1195.

Pachaly P, Schonhert6r-Weissbarth C and Sin KS (1990) New prenylflavonoid glycosides from *Epimedium koreanum*. *Planta Medica* **25**:277.

Parkin D, Pisani P and Ferlay J (1999) Global cancer statistics. CA: *A cancer journal for clinicians* **49**:33-64.

Perry LM and Metzger J (1980) *Medicinal Plants of East and Southeast Asia: Attributed Properties and Uses*, Cambridge.

Phani G, Gupta S, Murugan.M. P and Singh S (2009) Ethnobotanical Studies of Nubra Valley-A Cold Arid Zone of Himalaya. *Ethnobotanical Leaflets* **13**:752-765.

Prach K (1994).: Vegetation Succession on river gravel bars across the Northwestern Himalaya, *India Arctic & Alpine Research*, 26 (4) 349-353.

Qaiser M (1976) Flora of Pakistan. *Pak J Bot* **8** 199.

Qaiser M (1982) Tamaricaceae. In: Flora of Pakistan, E. Nasir and S.I. Ali, Rawalpindi.

# REFRENCES

Qaiser M and Perveen A (2004) Pollen Flora of Pakistan-XXXVII. Tamaricaceae. *Pak J Bot* **36**:1-18.

Qaiser M, Biosystematic Study of the family Tamaricaceae From Pakistan". PhD thesis, University of Karachi, Karachi. (1976) Biosystematic Study of the family Tamaricaceae From Pakistan, University of Karachi, Karachi.

Rice-Evans C, Miller N, Bolwell P, Bramley P and Pridh J (1995) The relative antioxidant activities of plant-derived polyphenolics and flavonoids. *Free Radical Res* **22**:375-383

Rios J and Puhalla S (2011) PARP inhibitors in breast cancer: BRCA and beyond. *Oncology* (Williston Park) **25**:1014-1025.

Said HM (1969) *Hamdard Pharmacopoeia of Eastern Medicines*, Pakistan.

Sakagami H, Jiang Y, Kusama K, Atsumi T, Ueha T, Toguchi M, Iwakura I, Satoh K, Ito H, Hatano T and Yoshida T (2000) Cytotoxic activity of hydrolyzable tannins against human oral tumor cell lines--a possible mechanism. *Phytomedicine* **7**:39–47.

Satoh M and Lindahl T (1992) Role of poly (ADP-ribose) formation in DNA repair. *Nature* **356**:356-358.

sheet F (1996) Twelve major cancers. *Scientific Am* **275**:92-98.

Skehan P, R. S, Scudiero D, Monks A and McMahon J (1990) New colorimetric cytotoxicity assay for anticancer-drug screening. *J Natl Cancer Inst* **82**:1107-1112.

Skehan P, Storeng R, Scudiero D, Monks A, McMahon J, Vistica D, Warren JT, Bokesch H, Kenney S and Boyd MR (1990) New colorimetric cytotoxicity assay for anticancer-drug screening. *J Natl Cancer Inst* **82**:1107-1112.

Smith I (1976) *Chromatographic and electrophoretic techniques*, fourth edition, Heinman, london. .

Smolarz H, Budzianowski J, Bogucka-Kocka A, Kocki J and Mendyk E (2008) Flavonoid glucuronides with anti-leukaemic activity from *Polygonum amphibium* L. *Phytochem Anal* **19**:506-513.

Sokolov LD (1986) *Rastitelnye USSR.*, USSR.

Song N, Xu W, Guan X, Wang.Y and Nie X (2007) Several flavonoids from *Capsella bursa-pastoris* (L.) Medic. *Asian Journal of Traditional Medicines* **2**:218-222.

Souleman A, Barakat H, Hussein S, El-Mousallamy A and Nawwar M (1998) Unique phenolic sulphate conjugates from the flowers of *Tamarix amplixuicaulis*. *Natural Product Sciences* **4**: 245-252

# REFRENCES

Swain T, Harborne JB and Van Sumere CF (1977) Biochemistry of Plant Phenolics, Plenum Press, New York.

Szaever H, Kaczmarek J, Rybczynska M and Baer-Dubowska W (2006) The effect of plant phenols on the expression and activity of phorbol ester-induced PKC in mousse epidermis. *Toxicology* **230**:1-10.

Takeya K and Itokawa H (1988) Chemical studies on the constituents of *Hyphear tanakae* Hosokawa from different host trees. *Chem Pharm Bull* **36**:1180-1184.

Thornes RD and O' Kennedy R (1997) Coumarins: biology, applications and mode of action, Jone Wiley and Sons, London.

Tomas-Barberan F, Iniesta – Sanmartin E, Ferreres F, Tomas – Lorente F, Trowitzsch-Kienasrt W and Wrayt V (1990) *Trans* – coniferyl alcohol 4- *O*-sulphated and flavonoid sulphates from some *Tamarix* species. *Phytochemistry* **29**:3050-3051.

Trease GE (1966) *Textbook of pharmacognosy*, Eighth Edition.

Urbatsch LE, Mabry TJ, Miyakado M, Ohno N and Yoshioka H (1976) Flavonol methyl ethers from *Ericameria diffusa*. *Phytochemistry* **15**:440.

Vichai V and Kirtikara K Sulforhodamine B colorimetric assay for cytotoxicity screening. *Nat Protoc* **1**:1112-1116.

Vogel AI (2001) *Text Book of Practical Organic Chemistry*, Furniss, B. S. and Hannaford,A . J. (E d s .), Longman Sceintific, New York.

Wang CC, Chen LG and Yang LL (1999) Antitumor activity of four macrocyclic ellagitannins from *Cuphea hyssopifolia*. *Cancer Lett* **140**:195–200.

Wang Y, Li H, Zhang G, Zhang Y and Chen L (2011) Traditional chinese medicine composition for treating insufficiency in cerebral blood supply. *Faming Zhuanli Shenqing*

WR Sykes & Williams PA (1999): *Myricaria germanica* (Tamaricaceae) wild in New Zealand (PDF, 2.1 MB). *New Zealand Botanical Society Newsletter*, **55**: 12-14, Christchurch.

Yamamoto Y, Ohara N, Ai CQ and Sugimoto K (2007a) Prophylactic and therapeutic compositions for fatigue containing herbal drugs and food and beverages containing the compositions. *Jpn Kokai Tokkyo Koho*.

Yamamoto Y, Ohara N, Ai CQ and Sugimoto K (2007b) skin external preparation with moisture keeping or skin roughness improving effect. *Jpn Kokai Tokkyo Koho*.

Yang L, Jiang H, Wang Q, Yang B and Kuang H (2012) A new feruloyl tyramine glycoside from the roots of *Achyranthes bidentata*. *Chin J Nat Med* **10**:16-19.

# REFERENCES

Yang LL, Lee CY and Yen KY (2000) Induction of apoptosis by hydrolyzable tannins from *Eugenia jambos* L. on human leukemia cells. *Cancer Lett* **157**:65–75.

Yang LL, Wang CC, Yen K, Yoshida T, Hatano T and Okuda T (2000b) Antitumor activities of ellagitannins on tumor cell lines. *Basic Life Sciences* **22**:615-628

Yang Q and Gaskin J (2007) Tamaricaceae in Flora of China, Beijing and St. Louis, Science Press and Missouri Botanical Garden Press.

Yasukawa K and Takido M (1987) A falvonol glycoside from *Lysimachia mauritiana*. *Phytochemistry* **26**:1224.

Yoshida T, Ahemad AF and Okuda T (1993a) Part III: New diimeric hydrolyzable tannins from *Reaumuria hirtella*. *Chem Pharm Bull* **41**:672-679.

Yoshida T, Ahemad AF, Memon MU and Okuda T (1991a) Part II :New Monomeric and Dimeric Hydrolyzable Tannins from *Reaumuria hirtella* and *Tamarix pakistanica*. *Chem Pharm Bull* **39**:2849-2854.

Yoshida T, Ahmed AF, Memon MU and Okuda T (1993b) dimeric hydrolysable tannins from *Tamarix pakistanica*. *Phytochemistry* **33**:197–202.

Yoshida T, Hatano T, Ahemad AF, Okonogi A and Okuda T (1991b) PartI: Structures of isorugosin E and Hirtellin B, dimeric hydrolysable tannins having a trisgalloyl group. *Tetrahedron* **47**:3575-3584.

Yoshida T, Hatano T, Ito H and Okuda T (2000) *Bioactive Natural Products*, Elsevier Science B.V.

Yoshida T, Hatano T, Ito H and Okuda T (2009) *Chemistry and Biology of Ellagitannins: An Underestimated Class of Bioactive Plant Polyphenols*, World Scientific Publishing, Singapore.

Yoshizawa S, Horiuchi T, Fujiki H, Yoshida T, Okuda T and Sugimura T (1987) Antitumor promoting activity of (-)-epigallocachechine gallate, the main constituent of "Tannins" in green tee. *Phytotherapy Res* **1**:44.

Yoshizawa S, Horiuchi T, Suganuma M, Nishiwaki S, Yatsunami J, Okabe S, Okuda T, Muro Y, Frenkel K, Troll W and Fujiki H (1992) Penta-O-galloyl-$\beta$-D-glucose and (-)-epigallocatechin gallate, in Phenolic Compounds in Food and Their Effects on Health II pp 316-325

Zhang J (2005) A patch for treating tumor and its preparation method. *Faming Zhuanli Shenqing*.

# REFRENCES

Zhang Q, Zhu J, Zhang Y, Chen L and Zhang G (2011a) Tibetan medicine composition containing Lamiophlomis and Oxytropis and others for treating bone fracture. *Faming Zhuanli Shenqing*.

Zhang T, Zhao Y, Cao Q, Hou J and Huang J (2012) Quality control method of Chinese medicinal preparation Wuweiganlu. *Faming Zhuanli Shenqing*.

Zhang X, Li Q, He R, Motwani M and Vasiliou V (2011) Synergistic inhibition of hepatocellular carcinoma growth by cotargeting chromatin modifying enzymes and poly (ADP-ribose) polymerases. *Hepatology* **55**:1840 - 1851.

Zhang Y, Yuan Y, Cui B and Li S (2011b) [Study on chemical constituents from ethyl acetate extract of *Myricaria bracteata*]. *Zhongguo Zhong yao za zhi = Zhongguo zhongyao zazhi = China journal of Chinese materia medica* **36**:1019-1023.

Zhao DB, Liu XH, Cui SY, Wang T and Wang HQ (2005a) Separation and determination of six active components in two *Myricaria* plants by capillary chromatography. *Chromatographia* **61**:643-646.

Zhou R, Wang T and Du XZ (2006) [Studies on chemical constituents in herb of *Myricaria bracteata*]. *Zhongguo Zhong yao za zhi = Zhongguo zhongyao zazhi = China journal of Chinese materia medica* **31**:474-476.

Zunino F and Capranico G (1997) *Cancer Therapeutics: Experimental and Clinical Agents, Cancer Drug Discovery and Development*; Humana Press: Totowa, Japan.

Zunino F and Capranico G (1997) *Cancer Therapeutics: Experimental and Clinical Agents, Cancer Drug Discovery and Development*; Humana Press: Totowa, Japan.

# APPENDIX

## Effect against PC3 prostate cell line

Crude Ext

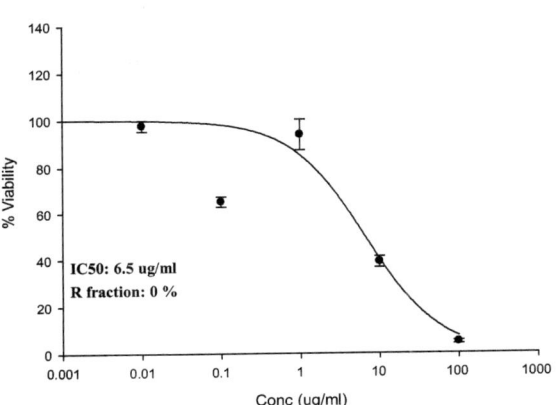

F-1

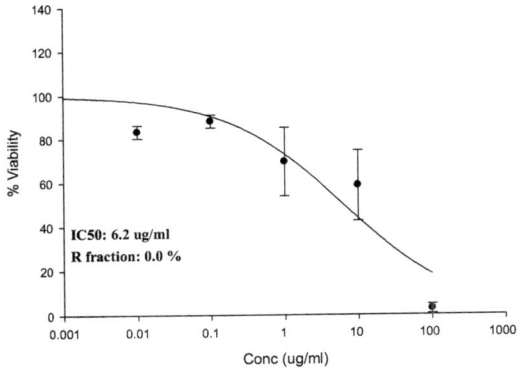

F-2

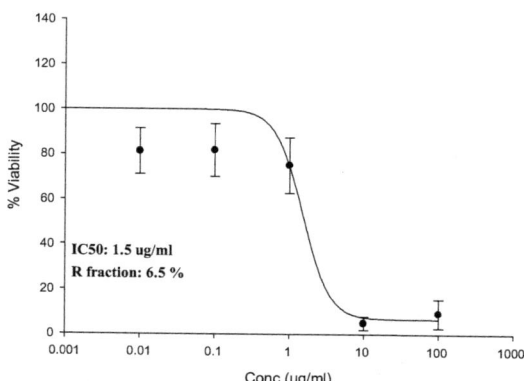

F-3

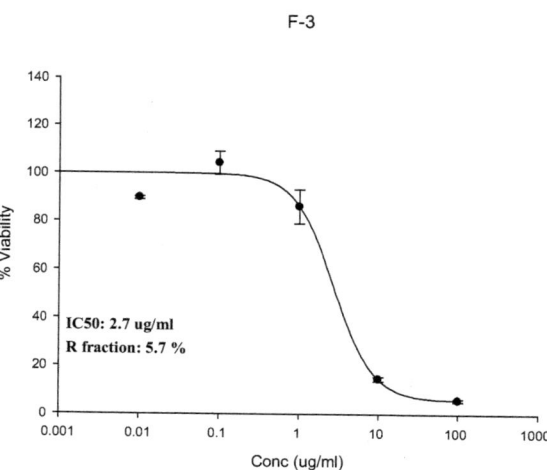

F-4

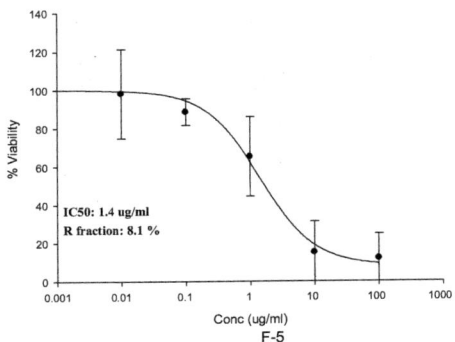

F-5

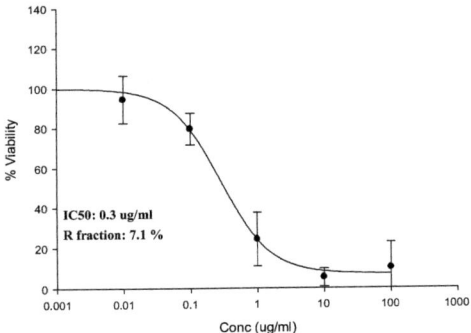

F-6

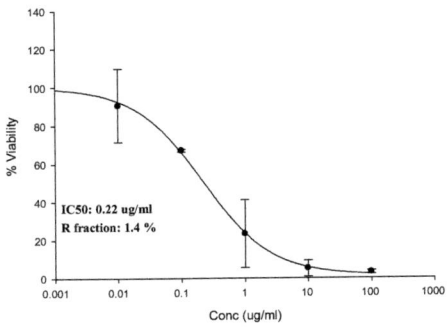

F-7

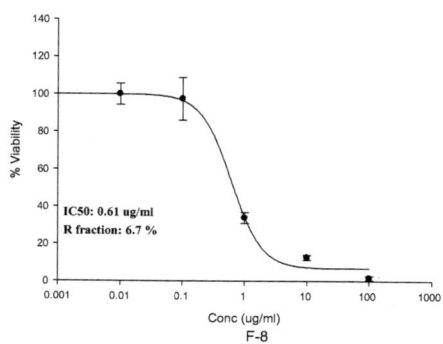

F-8

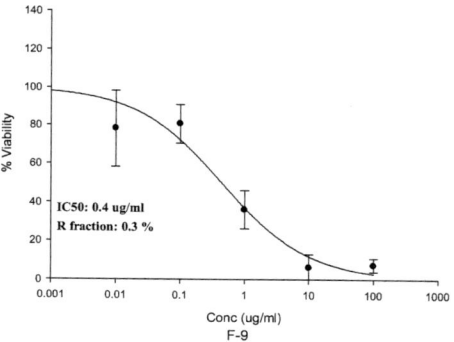

F-9

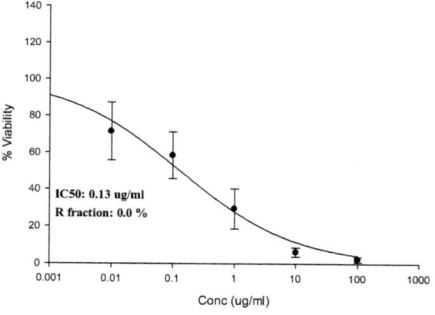

F-10

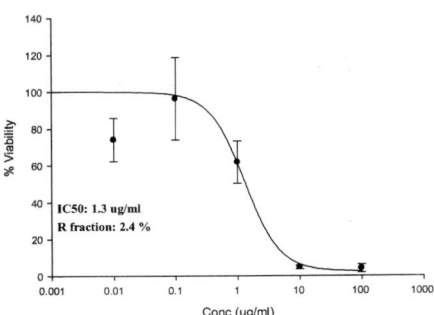

F-11

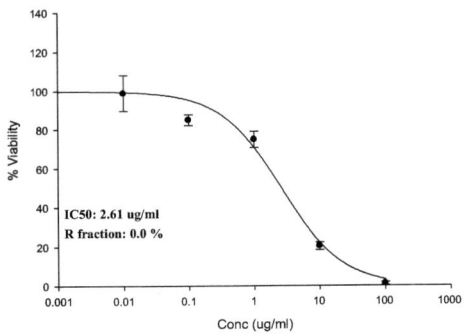

**Effect against Huh-7 liver cancer cell line**

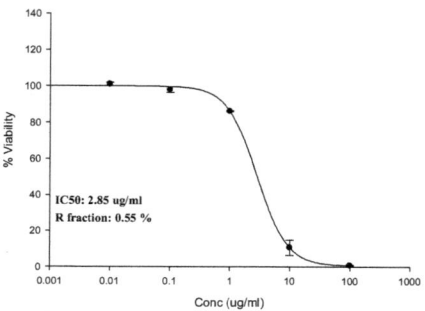

Crude ext

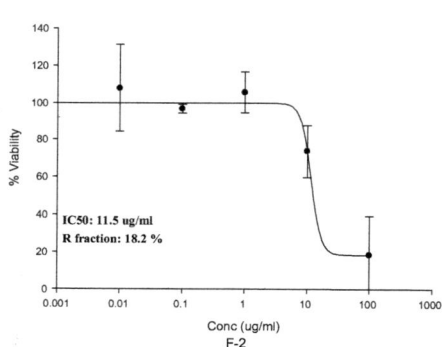

F-1

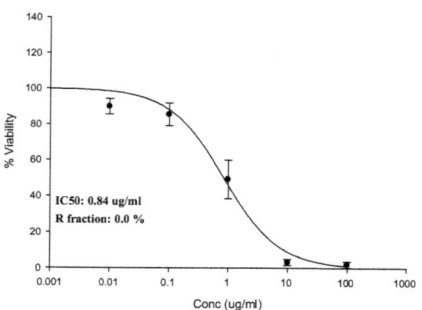

F-2

F-3

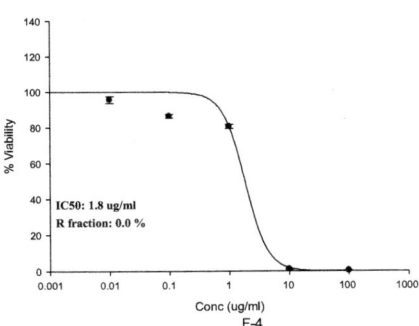

F-4

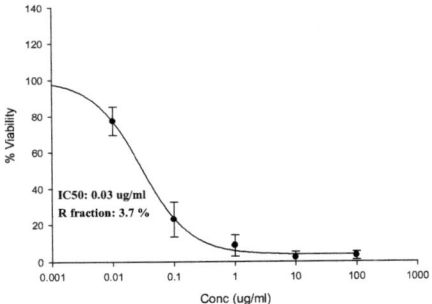

F-5

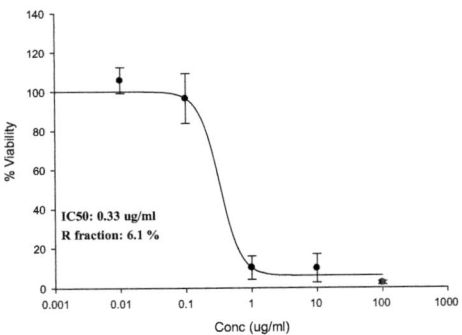

F-6

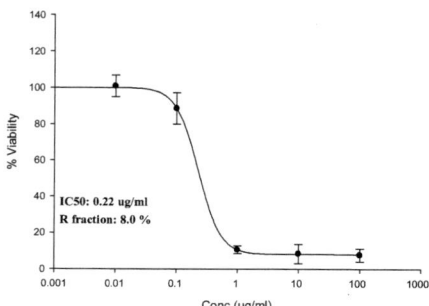

F-7

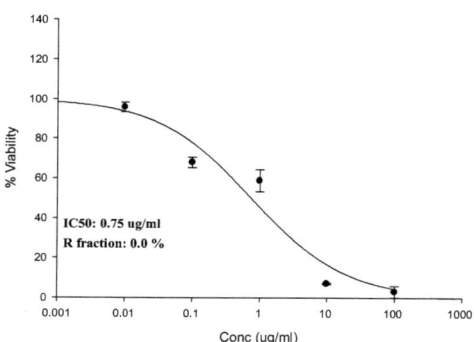

F-8

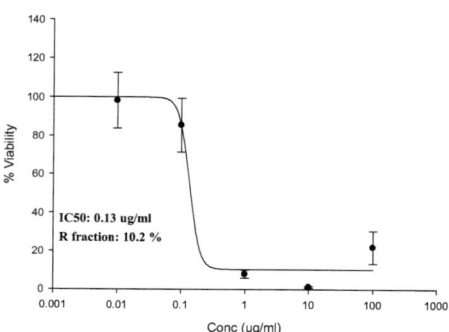

F-9

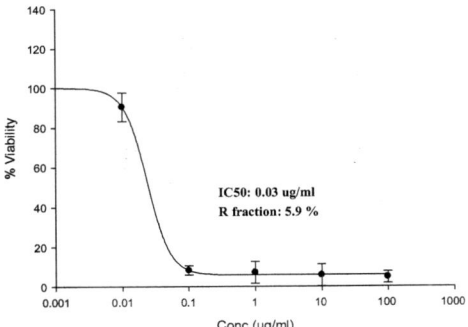

F-10

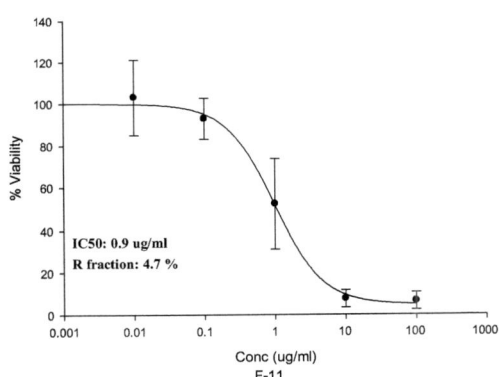

F-11

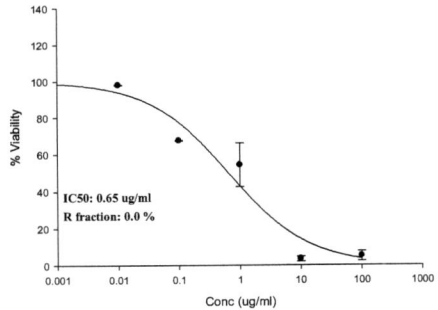

F-12

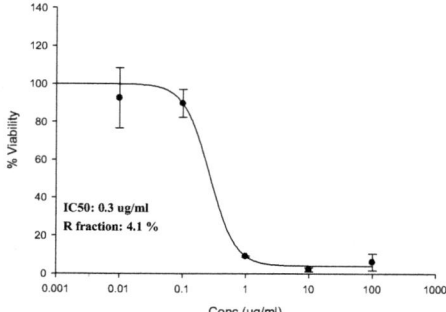

## Effect against MCF-7 breast cancer cell line

Crude Ext

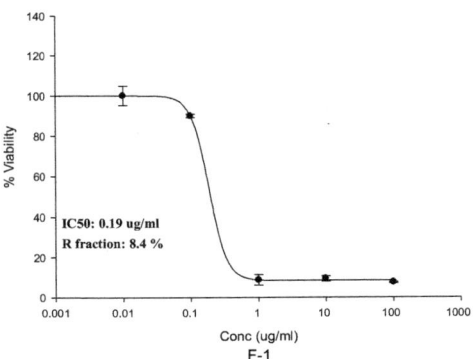

F-1

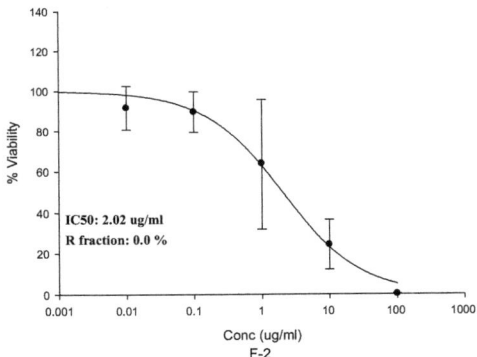

F-2

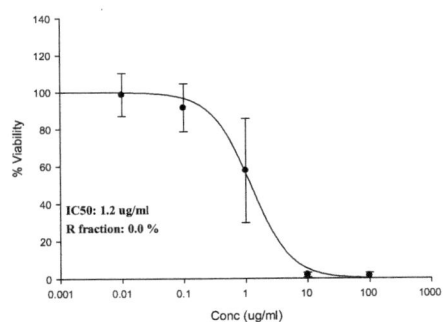

F-3

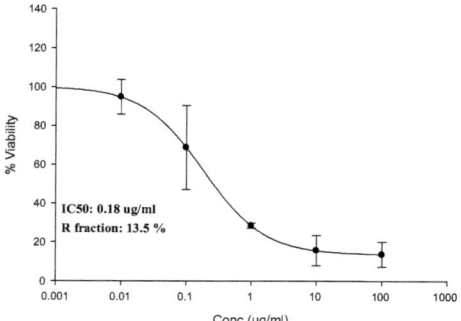

F-4

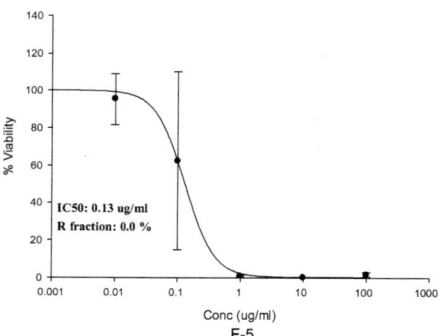

F-5

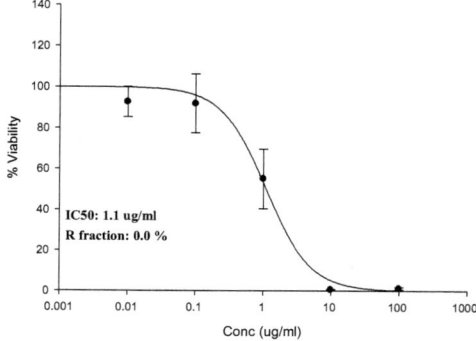

F-6

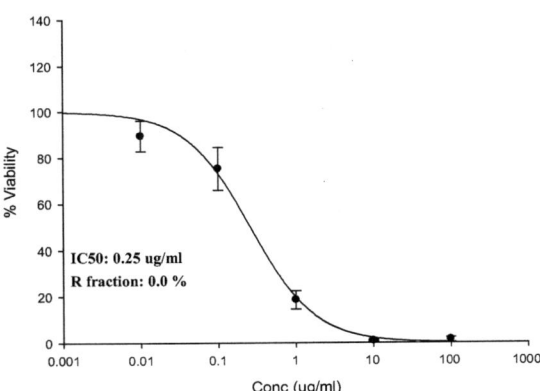

F-7

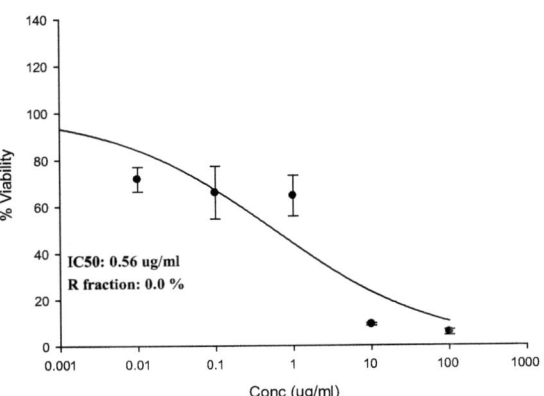

F-8

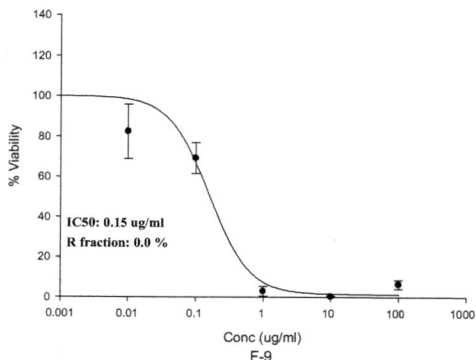

F-9

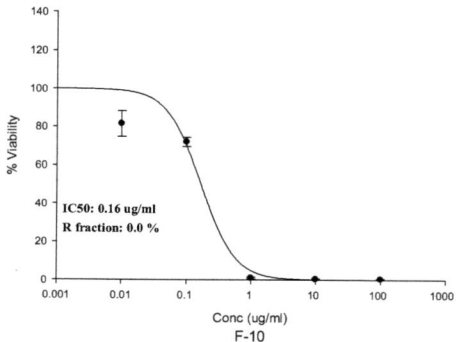

F-10

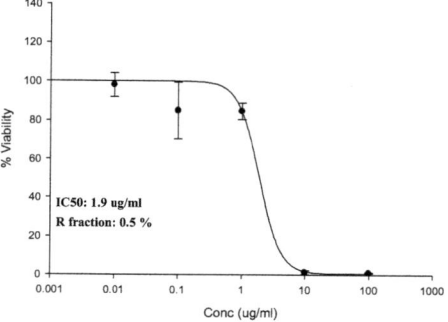

F-11

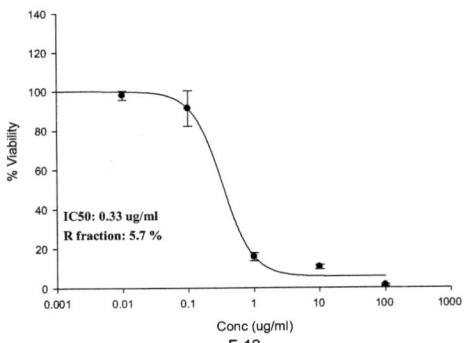

F-12

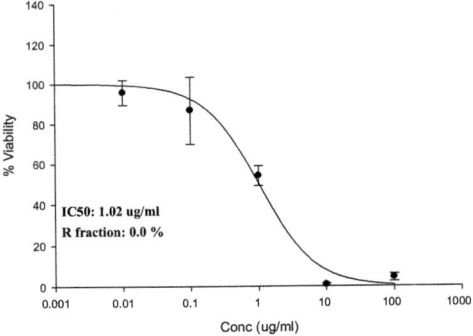

# ACKNOWLEDGEMENTS

I would like to express my gratitude and appreciation to the following people who significantly contributed to the work done in this thesis:

Prof. Dr. Ulrike Lindequist, Institut für Pharmazie, Lehrstuhl für Pharmazeutische Biologie, Ernst-Moritz-Arndt Universität, Greifswald, Germany, for her kind support and unremitting encouragement throughout my PhD and of course for her supervising, constructive criticism, sound advices and great effort in revising the thesis.

Prof. Dr. Mahmoud A. M. Nawwar, Professor of Phytochemistry, National Research Centre, NRC, Cairo, for his continuous scientific guidance, valuable discussions, helpful suggestions, generous support, specially the NMR interpretation and extensive efforts throughout this thesis.

I would like to thank the colleagues of the Botanical gardens of the Universities Bonn and Regensburg for the friendly providing of plant material of *Myricaria germanica* and PD Dr. Peter König, Botanical garden, University Greifswald, for intermediation and taxonomic authentication

Prof. Dr. Ashraf Abdel Naiem, Prof. of Pharmacology and Toxicology, Faculty of Pharmacy, Ain-Shams University, Cairo, Egypt for his essential assistance, valuable guidance and constructive criticism especially for the cytotoxicity assessment.

I am thankful to all my colleagues at the NRC and Greifswald, for their cooperation, encouragement and support. I esteemed their honesty and constructive criticism.

I would like to express my deepest gratitude to my parents and my brother especially my mum for her fruitful contribution with important advices and support during this thesis.
Finally, I would like to thank my husband and my son Adam for their boundless love, encouragement, support and most for their patience.

Noha Swilam

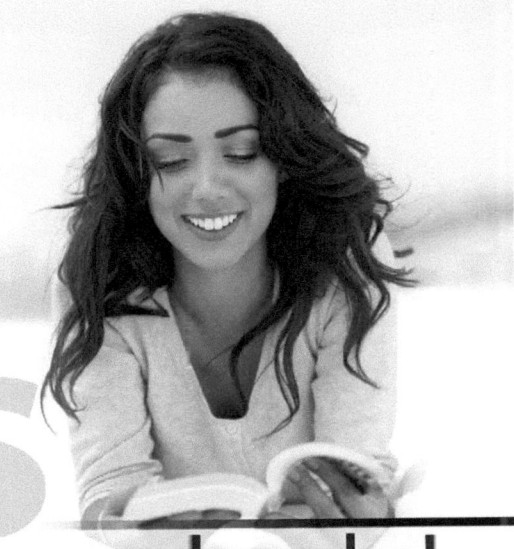

# i want morebooks!

Buy your books fast and straightforward online - at one of the world's fastest growing online book stores! Environmentally sound due to Print-on-Demand technologies.

Buy your books online at
# www.get-morebooks.com

Kaufen Sie Ihre Bücher schnell und unkompliziert online – auf einer der am schnellsten wachsenden Buchhandelsplattformen weltweit!
Dank Print-On-Demand umwelt- und ressourcenschonend produziert.

Bücher schneller online kaufen
# www.morebooks.de

OmniScriptum Marketing DEU GmbH
Heinrich-Böcking-Str. 6-8
D - 66121 Saarbrücken
Telefax: +49 681 93 81 567-9

info@omniscriptum.de
www.omniscriptum.de

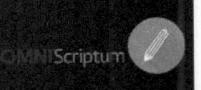

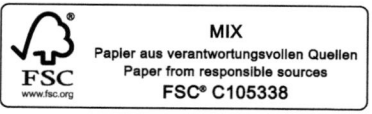

Printed by Books on Demand GmbH, Norderstedt / Germany